Politics in the Making of HIV/AIDS in South Africa

Politics in the Making of HIV/AIDS in South Africa

Kiran Pienaar
Curtin University, Australia

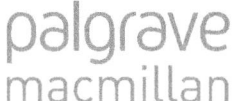

© Kiran Pienaar 2016

All rights reserved. No reproduction, copy or transmission of this publication may be made without written permission.

No portion of this publication may be reproduced, copied or transmitted save with written permission or in accordance with the provisions of the Copyright, Designs and Patents Act 1988, or under the terms of any licence permitting limited copying issued by the Copyright Licensing Agency, Saffron House, 6–10 Kirby Street, London EC1N 8TS.

Any person who does any unauthorized act in relation to this publication may be liable to criminal prosecution and civil claims for damages.

The author has asserted her right to be identified as the author of this work in accordance with the Copyright, Designs and Patents Act 1988.

First published 2016 by
PALGRAVE MACMILLAN

Palgrave Macmillan in the UK is an imprint of Macmillan Publishers Limited, registered in England, company number 785998, of Houndmills, Basingstoke, Hampshire RG21 6XS.

Palgrave Macmillan in the US is a division of St Martin's Press LLC, 175 Fifth Avenue, New York, NY 10010.

Palgrave Macmillan is the global academic imprint of the above companies and has companies and representatives throughout the world.

Palgrave® and Macmillan® are registered trademarks in the United States, the United Kingdom, Europe and other countries.

ISBN 978–1–137–50500–2

This book is printed on paper suitable for recycling and made from fully managed and sustained forest sources. Logging, pulping and manufacturing processes are expected to conform to the environmental regulations of the country of origin.

A catalogue record for this book is available from the British Library.

Library of Congress Cataloging-in-Publication Data
Names: Pienaar, Kiran, 1983–, author.
Title: Politics in the making of HIV/AIDS in South Africa / Kiran Pienaar.
Description: Basingstoke, Hampshire ; New York, NY : Palgrave Macmillan, 2016. | Includes bibliographical references and index.
Identifiers: LCCN 2015029312 | ISBN 9781137505002 (hardback)
Subjects: | MESH: Acquired Immunodeficiency Syndrome—epidemiology—South Africa. | HIV Infections—epidemiology—South Africa. | Health Policy—South Africa. | Politics—South Africa. | Socioeconomic Factors—South Africa.
Classification: LCC RA643.86.S6 | NLM WC 503.4 HU5 | DDC 362.19697/9200968—dc23
LC record available at http://lccn.loc.gov/2015029312

Contents

Acknowledgements	vi
List of Abbreviations	viii
Introduction: HIV/AIDS as a Site of Struggle in South Africa	1
1 Disease in Theory and Practice	20
2 Contesting Science, Making Disease	35
3 Poverty in the Making of HIV/AIDS	67
4 Disease as a Politics of the Human	96
Conclusion: Towards an Ontological Politics of Disease	120
Appendix A: An Overview of the Struggles over HIV in South Africa (1998–2014)	135
Notes	141
Bibliography	145
Index	155

Acknowledgements

The trajectory this book has taken is in no small measure due to the incisive critique and guidance of Suzanne Fraser and Steven Angelides. I owe an enormous debt of gratitude to them as I recognise that without their thoughtful theoretical insights, this book would not have taken the shape it has and the task of writing it would not have been as rewarding. I am also grateful to Mark Davis, Marsha Rosengarten and Kane Race for their critical feedback, which encouraged me to clarify the arguments of the book.

For their unwavering support, love and care, I extend heartfelt thanks to my family. I also benefited from the encouragement, advice and remarkable generosity of my friends. I thank in particular Samantha Balaton-Chrimes for her steadfast friendship and immeasurable support over the years. I extend thanks to Rebecca Hodes and the staff at the AIDS Society Research Unit (ASRU) for hosting me during my fieldwork trip to South Africa.

The research on which this book is based would not have been possible without the financial support of two Monash University scholarships, an International Postgraduate Research Scholarship and a Graduate Scholarship.

Some of the material in this book has previously appeared in print. Sections of Chapter 2 have appeared in Pienaar, K. (2014), '(Re)reading the political conflict over HIV in South Africa (1999–2008): A new materialist analysis', *Social Theory & Health*, 12: 179–196. Parts of the argument in Chapter 4 have appeared in Pienaar, K. (2015) 'Claiming rights, making citizens: HIV and the performativity of biological citizenship', *Social Theory & Health*, early online, DOI 10.1057/sth.2015.26. This material is reprinted here with permission of Macmillan Publishers Ltd.

Finally, special thanks to Bradley Clayton for sharing and delighting in 'all the things', not least many Saturday morning discussions on posthumanism and new materialist approaches. I am especially grateful for your countless acts of kindness and love that sustained me throughout this project. Words are inadequate to express my gratitude to you.

This inevitably partial list is testament to the extent to which intellectual interlocutors, family, friends, academic institutions, departments, institutional spaces, and many more ('human' and 'non-human') participants have helped constitute this book. I gratefully acknowledge all those entangled with this work who, in different and important ways, have enabled it to emerge.

Abbreviations

AIDS	Acquired immune deficiency syndrome
ANC	African National Congress
ART	Anti-retroviral therapy
ARV	Anti-retroviral
CD4	Cluster of Differentiation Four
DA	Democratic Alliance
DNA	Deoxyribonucleic acid
DOT-TB	Directly Observed Therapy for Tuberculosis
G8	Group of Eight
GRID	Gay related immune deficiency disease
HAART	Highly active anti-retroviral therapy
HIV	Human immunodeficiency virus
HSRC	Human Sciences Research Council
IAS	International AIDS Society
ID	Independent Democrats
IFP	Inkatha Freedom Party
MCC	Medicines Control Council
MP	Member of Parliament
MSF	Médecins Sans Frontières
NAPWA	National Association of People with AIDS
NGO	Non-governmental organisation
NSP	National Strategic Plan (on HIV)
Oxfam	Oxford Committee for Famine Relief
PMTCT	Prevention of mother-to-child transmission
PrEP	Pre-Exposure Prophylaxis
RNA	Ribonucleic acid
RSA	Republic of South Africa
STS	Science and Technology Studies
TAC	Treatment Action Campaign
TB	Tuberculosis
UDHR	Universal Declaration of Human Rights
UNAIDS	Joint United Nations Programme on HIV/AIDS
WHO	World Health Organization

Introduction: HIV/AIDS as a Site of Struggle in South Africa

Few issues define the new South Africa as forcefully as HIV/AIDS.[1] This is, of course, partly because South Africa has the largest HIV epidemic in the world (UNAIDS, 2012). However, it is also because HIV/AIDS has been a major source of conflict in post-apartheid South Africa, generating a series of public disputes and legal battles between the fledgling democratic government and local civil society organisations. The conflict is closely connected to former president Thabo Mbeki's views on HIV/AIDS. Mbeki famously challenged the scientific orthodoxy, insisting that AIDS is a disease of poverty and not simply the outcome of a viral infection. As he put it:

> The world's biggest killer and the greatest cause of ill health and suffering across the globe, including South Africa, is extreme poverty [...] As I listened and heard the whole story told about our own country, it seemed to me that we could not blame everything on a single virus [HIV]. (Mbeki, 2000d)

In response, local HIV activists (such as Geffen quoted below), endorsed the prevailing scientific view, arguing that while poverty contributes to the disease, AIDS is caused by a viral infection: 'Only HIV predicts AIDS [...] No other factor on its own, including drug use, diet or poverty, is sufficient to cause AIDS' (Geffen, 2006). It is, of course, possible to understand AIDS as causally related both to a viral infection and to poverty. However, I suggest that if we are to understand the dynamic and emergent character of AIDS, both conceptions prove insufficient as they reduce disease to a matter of fact: a fixed object that is either the product of biological forces (a viral infection) or the product of social forces (poverty). Disease, as this book seeks to show, exceeds any notion of simple fact, whether facts are construed as effects of biological or social factors. Indeed, the complexities of HIV/AIDS in South Africa and the continually changing character of the epidemic point to the need for a new conceptual approach, one which treats the facts of disease as temporary and contingent, rather than stable and foundational.

This book is a modest attempt to respond to this need. It offers a theoretically nuanced and empirically grounded analysis of HIV/AIDS in South Africa, addressing in particular the generative role of politics in producing the disease and its facts. Importantly, and in contrast to the conventional view of disease as a fixed entity, possessed of intrinsic characteristics, the analysis proceeds from the premise that disease is always under construction, its characteristics forged through, rather than preceding, political and social forces. The book maps some of these forces in the context of the South African epidemic, showing how they have helped to constitute HIV/AIDS in specific and often harmful ways. For example, it examines the role of state–civil society conflict, poverty, specific health promotion strategies and colonial-apartheid public health policies in producing ontologies of HIV/AIDS unique to South Africa. By tracking the practices and processes through which HIV/AIDS has been variously constituted, the book seeks to persuade readers that there is nothing natural or inevitable about the character of the disease in South Africa. Disease and its effects can always be made differently. It is this insight about the open-endedness of disease that not only distinguishes this book from other social studies of HIV in South Africa but also opens up new, fruitful avenues for addressing the epidemic. But before exploring these ideas about the ontology of disease any further, it is necessary to give some background to the politics of HIV in South Africa by sketching the contestation over the science of HIV that occurred under the Mbeki government.

South Africa's struggle over the science of HIV

An estimated 5.6 million people live with HIV in South Africa, making the country's HIV-positive population the biggest in the world (UNAIDS, 2012). Although the number of new infections is declining as the epidemic levels off, it remains very high with approximately 1284 South Africans newly infected with HIV each day (Shisana *et al.*, 2014). Corresponding to the high rates of infection, the International AIDS Society (2009) estimates that almost 1000 AIDS-related deaths occur in South Africa every day. Yet, it was only in 2003 – 21 years after the first cases of HIV were diagnosed in South Africa – that the national government announced its commitment to a comprehensive treatment programme to address the country's severe epidemic. The delay in delivering a national treatment programme is connected to the AIDS dissident response of South Africa's second democratically elected leader, former president Thabo Mbeki. It is Mbeki's AIDS dissidence and its effects – as part of the politics of HIV/AIDS in South Africa – that is the focus of this book.

Often characterised as an 'AIDS denialist', Mbeki is perhaps most wellknown for questioning the viral causation of AIDS and for disputing the efficacy of biomedical treatment. He publicly challenged mainstream (Western) science on HIV and called for an African response to the 'uniquely African catastrophe' of HIV, not 'a simple superimposition of Western experience on African reality' (Mbeki, 2000c). In June 2000, less than a year after he was elected president, Mbeki convened a panel of mainstream and dissident scientists to review the science on HIV/AIDS, including whether HIV causes AIDS (Schneider, 2002). The dissident and orthodox scientists on the panel were unable to reach agreement on the putative causes and treatment of the disease. They engaged in a public dispute, culminating in the dissident panellists issuing a 'Minority Statement', which contested the link between HIV and AIDS and asserted that anti-retroviral (ARV) drugs – the best-known medical treatment for HIV – are 'killing people' (Bialy et al., 2000, para. 4). Meanwhile, the other members of the panel launched an international petition in support of mainstream HIV science (Schneider, 2002). This petition, known as the 'Durban Declaration' (2000), was signed by 5000 scientists and presented at the Thirteenth International AIDS conference, held in Durban, South Africa in July 2000.

As may be clear from the contestation between members of the AIDS advisory panel, Mbeki's dissident views were not widely shared, but they were endorsed by a small, powerful group of loyalists in the ruling African National Congress (ANC), including the then Health Minister, Mantombazana Tshabalala-Msimang (Youdé, 2007a). Like Mbeki, Tshabalala-Msimang was sceptical about the efficacy of ARVs, raising concerns about their toxicity and potentially harmful long-term impact. Because of these concerns, she expressed reluctance to adopt a public sector anti-retroviral therapy (ART) programme, stressing instead the value of an HIV policy that focused on prevention (ced Tshabalala-Msimang, 2004).[2] Mbeki and Tshabalala-Msimang were, of course, not solely responsible for South Africa's policy approach to HIV/AIDS but their dissident views, along with those of their policy advisors, helped to shape the national response to HIV during Mbeki's presidency and in the succeeding years (Youdé, 2007a). Fortunately, the era of AIDS dissidence in South Africa is now over but, as this book reveals, it has shaped the contours and effects of the HIV epidemic in that country in significant ways.

Given Mbeki's role in shaping South Africa's HIV policy and his expressed scepticism of mainstream science on HIV (Youdé, 2005), it is perhaps not surprising that his dissident views were publicly challenged by South African civil society, notably by prominent local HIV/AIDS organisation, the Treatment Action Campaign (TAC). With more than 16,000 members and 276 branches countrywide, the TAC is the largest South African non-governmental organisation (NGO) for people living with HIV (Peacock et al., 2008). As the most vocal critic of the Mbeki executive's approach to HIV, the TAC launched a civil disobedience campaign to protest the absence of a national HIV treatment plan (Heywood, 2004). The campaign included protests, marches, pickets and laying a charge of culpable homicide against the Minister of Health for her decision not to deliver a government-funded ART programme (Low et al., 2010). The TAC's resistance to the government's HIV policy was not confined to civil disobedience tactics and public protests, however; the organisation also took legal action against the government for its failure to develop a national programme for the prevention of mother-to-child transmission of HIV (PMTCT). TAC leaders resorted to litigation in August 2001 after the government refused to increase access to PMTCT in the public health care system, citing concerns about the toxicity of the ARV drugs used for PMTCT (Heywood, 2003).

Although other civil society organisations also contested the government's approach to HIV, the TAC was 'the only organisation prepared to robustly and unapologetically challenge AIDS denialism, thus souring relations between TAC, the ANC [African National Congress] and the Ministry of Health' (Heywood, 2004, p. 13). The TAC's most public challenge to the Mbeki government's AIDS dissidence occurred at the 2006 International AIDS conference in Toronto. South Africa's stand at the conference featured a controversial display of lemons, garlic and beetroot, which Health Minister Tshabalala-Msimang endorsed as nutritional remedies for HIV (Kapp, 2006). TAC members occupied the stand, protesting the prominence it gave to nutritional remedies at the expense of ART. Later, in a plenary session at the conference, executive TAC member Mark Heywood called for the health minister's immediate dismissal (Low et al., 2010). In 2008, Mbeki stepped down as president and since then TAC has enjoyed more cooperative relations with the

Introduction 5

two post-Mbeki governments (Mbali, 2013). However, the legacy of the TAC–government conflict endures in the uneven distribution of South Africa's HIV epidemic and the damaging effects of his government's delay in delivering HIV treatment.

Given that the TAC was the major countervailing voice in civil society, openly challenging the government's AIDS dissidence, the organisation's position on HIV presents a useful point of comparison to that of the government and, more generally, the TAC–government conflict presents an obvious choice for examining the negotiations and struggles over HIV in South Africa. By way of background, I have mapped some of these struggles and the associated actions of both the government and TAC in the timeline provided as Appendix A. This timeline depicts the orthodox view of the TAC–government conflict, outlining its apparent form and effects. The book problematises this view, querying the commonplace assumption that the conflict exists separately from and posterior to HIV. Focusing on the periods coinciding with Mbeki's two terms of office (1999–2008) and the scale-up of ART in South Africa (2004–12), it examines how the TAC–government dispute over HIV helped to materially shape the disease and, in turn, the epidemic. It argues that the dispute itself is part of the politics that makes HIV as disease, constituting it in ways unique to South Africa. In making this argument, the book addresses a broader set of concerns about the ontology of disease that owe much to the theoretical insights of Science and Technology Studies (STS) and feminist theory:

- Disease is not a static, immutable object. It is emergent and dynamic and, as such, is always open to change.
- Disease does not precede human action. Rather it is made and remade within it.
- Human actions alone do not make disease; it is through the encounters of humans and non-humans that disease is forged and changed.
- Disease is politics: it is a site of, and emerges through, ongoing political negotiation and contestation. To put this slightly differently, disease is politically constructed, but no less real for being thus constructed.

Before explaining these theoretical concerns in more detail, I turn next to the existing scholarship on the South African HIV debate, outlining the openings in the literature that form the point of departure for this book.

Rethinking the politics of HIV under Mbeki

The issue of government-led AIDS dissidence (or 'denialism') has attracted considerable scholarly attention, perhaps because it is associated with the rejection of proven medical treatments for HIV and is perceived to lead to preventable deaths. Most of the existing research on the Mbeki government's AIDS dissidence presents political analyses of the major events, statements and policy decisions in the state–civil society conflict on HIV/AIDS, drawing attention to the political and historical forces shaping the conflict (for example, Decoteau, 2008; Fassin, 2007; Gumede, 2005; van der Vliet, 2004). Much of the existing scholarship seeks to explain the rationale or underlying motivation for the Mbeki government's unique response to HIV (see, for example, Fourie and Meyer, 2010; Mbali, 2004; Schneider and Fassin, 2002). In this vein, Mbali (2004) argues that Mbeki's AIDS dissidence was motivated by his opposition to Western biomedicine and his belief that AIDS is a disease of poverty. Meanwhile, Schneider (2002) proposes that although the conflict was ostensibly about the causation of AIDS and appropriate treatment strategies, it was actually a struggle between the new government and civil society over the right to contribute to knowledge and exercise oversight in policy formation. Other research has also addressed the politics of knowledge at work in the South African struggle over HIV. In a book on the subject, Youdé (2007a, p. 123) draws on the concept of the 'epistemic community' to argue that, by challenging the scientific orthodoxy, the Mbeki government created a 'counter-epistemic community [that...] reinforces South Africa's negative past experiences with public health interventions and its desire to foster an African Renaissance-inspired identity'. This argument locates the Mbeki government's AIDS dissidence in South Africa's colonial-apartheid history and its desire to encourage African political autonomy and self-reliance by finding local solutions to the HIV epidemic.

While these studies offer very helpful accounts of the politics of HIV/AIDS in South Africa and illuminate the historical context of Mbeki's AIDS dissidence, they leave open a key question: how has AIDS dissidence helped to materially shape the disease in South Africa? This question may have been overlooked by existing research because of a tendency to treat understandings of disease (including dissident ones) as separate from the disease itself. On this view, theories or 'ideas about disease' are taken to be representative of, and therefore distinct from, the 'underlying reality of disease'. Although the assumption of a theory–reality split is commonplace in accounts of disease (Treichler, 1999), it obscures the generative role of theory, concepts and ideas in actually constituting disease. My aim in this book is to complicate the distinction between 'ideas about HIV/AIDS' (theory) and the 'disease itself' (reality), and in doing so propose a rethinking of HIV/AIDS in the context of South Africa. In place of the familiar view of HIV/AIDS as a fixed object that pre-exists our attempts to know it, I proceed on the conviction that ideas about HIV/AIDS – including dissident ones – and the reality of the disease are reciprocally constituted: they make and change each other, even as each undergoes change. So instead of asking (as much of the existing research has done) *What is the rationale for AIDS dissidence and how does it (mis)represent the reality of the disease?*, this book addresses the question *How does AIDS dissidence help to materialise the disease?* In reorienting the direction of analysis in this way, the aim is to move beyond accounts that pit 'representation' against 'reality', and engage instead the performativity of particular ideas about HIV: how they shape the materiality of the disease in South Africa.

The question of performativity is an important one because it makes use of recent scholarly advances that illuminate the ways in which disease is forged through, rather than preceding, our attempts to know it (see, for example, the work of Rosengarten [2009] on HIV, Fraser and Seear [2011] on hepatitis C and Seear [2014] on endometriosis). Challenging the familiar view that we can apprehend an independently existing reality through the right theories and concepts, such scholarship proposes that theory is both of reality and partakes in its making. This reconceptualisation of the relationship between theory and reality is especially helpful in countering the possible criticism that research such as this, which examines understandings of disease, diverts attention away from the urgent, real-life effects of disease. As cultural studies scholar Paula Treichler puts it, in arguing for the role of theory in confronting the HIV epidemic, 'theory *is* about "people's lives"' (1999, p. 3, emphasis added). In an effort to shed light on the links between disease concepts (theory) and the materiality of disease, the book tracks how particular understandings of HIV help to make the disease and those living with it. So, for example, where poor people are stigmatised as the carriers of HIV, they may be driven underground and are less likely to access HIV prevention services. Thus, HIV rates may increase among this demographic, helping to (re)produce HIV as a disease of the poor. The key point here is that this enactment of HIV is not anterior to human action. Rather it is realised through our actions, including our efforts to understand and treat the disease. If disease is made through human actions and processes, when these change, so too does the very materiality of disease. In short, disease and its effects are not inevitable; they could always be otherwise. In the chapters that follow, I demonstrate the political purchase of this approach, arguing that it affords opportunities for reconstituting HIV and undoing the damaging effects of current enactments of the disease.

Before exploring these theoretical points further, I return briefly to the existing scholarship on the politics of HIV/AIDS in South Africa to elaborate on the openings in the literature to which this study responds. Beyond a tendency to treat AIDS dissidence as separate from the disease itself, much of the existing scholarship offers a synchronic analysis, focusing on the era of the Mbeki government's AIDS dissidence. Because of this focus, many studies have tended to neglect the significance of successive governments' inaction in shaping the contours and effects of the epidemic in South Africa. A notable exception to this trend is a monograph by South African scholars Pieter Fourie and Melissa Meyer (2010), entitled *The Politics of AIDS Denialism: South Africa's Failure to Respond*. The book situates the Mbeki government's response to HIV in the context of South Africa's history of government lethargy and vacillation in combating the epidemic. As a genealogy of the politics of HIV in South Africa, it serves as an important reminder that the Mbeki administration's dissident policy did not emerge in a historical vacuum; it was shaped by the former apartheid government's 'racist-moralist' policy approach and by the Mandela government's failure to prioritise HIV/AIDS (Fourie and Meyer, 2010, p. 173). However, because of its focus on government policy, the analysis pays only limited attention to civil society's response to the problem of HIV, outlining in broad terms the points of contestation between the two sectors. Yet, just as AIDS dissidence was forged in relation to successive government inaction, it was also forged through specific civil society responses. Addressing the important role of state–civil society relations in materialising HIV, this book compares the approach of the government with that of leading South African civil society organisation, the TAC, arguing that they understood the causes and treatment of AIDS in somewhat different, though not incommensurate ways. Because TAC and the government constituted the problem of HIV differently, each proposed different measures to address it, with rather mixed effects. As I will show, these measures jointly shaped HIV in South Africa, sometimes in ways that actually helped to intensify, rather than alleviate, the effects of the epidemic.

Also noteworthy in the aforementioned literature is a tendency to reinforce the apparent polarisation of the state–civil society struggle by characterising it as a battle between orthodox science and AIDS dissidence, between responsible HIV activists and an irresponsible, autocratic government. For example, in her analysis of Mbeki's AIDS dissidence, postcolonial scholar Joy Wang describes the conflict thus:

> [T]he wider debate on AIDS denialism has until now – with few exceptions – been characterised by total polarisation. On the one hand, a small panel of 'dissident' scientists [...] have legitimised and commended Mbeki's resistance against ARV treatment. On the other hand, critics such as [HIV activist] Edwin Cameron [...] have charged Mbeki with nothing less than genocide; for criminal inaction leading to the deaths of [...] thousands of South Africans [...] Mainstream debate has affirmed [Cameron's] critical stance, presenting AIDS activists as moral humanitarians in a frustrating deadlock with an ANC government prone to despotism, corruption and a total disregard for human rights. (Wang, 2004, p. 3)

By analysing the debate through the lenses of orthodox/dissident science and moral/immoral responses to HIV, existing research ends up implicitly endorsing conventional (positivist) science as 'truth' and relegating AIDS dissident theories to the realm of irresponsible pseudoscience. I suggest that a more complex dynamic exists between AIDS dissidence and science, a dynamic that is eclipsed by assuming they are necessarily polarised positions, which rely on divergent epistemologies. While my desire to complicate the absolute polarisation of science and pseudoscience is somewhat unusual in analyses of the South African HIV debate, it allows consideration of both the continuities *and* discontinuities between AIDS dissident and scientific accounts, and indeed prompts the recognition that they are mutually constituted. Moreover, the analysis reveals that the presumed polarisation of the debate shaped HIV itself, enabling certain enactments of the disease to emerge, and ruling out others. It is only through a careful mapping of the enactments of HIV produced (and foreclosed) by the debate that it becomes possible to consider how HIV/AIDS might be made differently, in ways that move beyond the tenacious dualisms of orthodoxy/dissidence and science/pseudoscience.

Disease in the making: the turn to a materialist mode

To make the argument that HIV in South Africa has been materially shaped by the state–civil society conflict and its aftermath, I draw on an emerging theoretical literature about the ontology of disease, one which understands disease as made in practice and therefore as open to being remade. Central to this understanding is the work of ethnographer and philosopher Annemarie Mol (2002), who argues that disease, like all phenomena, is constantly in the making. Mol calls her approach *praxiography* to articulate her interest in the practices that make disease. The theoretical concepts underpinning Mol's approach are discussed in more detail in Chapter 1, but for now it is sufficient to note that praxiography disrupts the conventional view of disease as a fixed, singular and stable object. Instead, it posits disease as ontologically multiple, variously enacted in daily practices across different sites, such as the hospital, the body and the laboratory:

> If we no longer presume 'disease' to be a universal object hidden under *the* body's skin, but make the praxiographic shift to studying bodies and diseases while they are being enacted in daily hospital practices, multiplication follows. In practice a disease [...] is no longer *one*. (Mol, 2002, p. 83, emphasis in the original)

This radical refiguring of the ontology of disease has a number of significant implications. It enables an examination of the generative role of political and scientific practices in making disease – here practices are understood not as neutral mechanisms for intervening to 'address' disease but as directly shaping its very substance. Importantly, the approach Mol elaborates challenges the familiar conception of disease and its subjects as naturally given entities, which possess certain immutable attributes. Applied to HIV, this means that the materiality of the disease, and those living with it, is constantly under construction, rather than given in nature and fixed. For example, it is neither natural nor inevitable that young black women aged 17 to 34 have the highest rates of HIV infection in South Africa. As the analysis conducted in Chapter 2 reveals, this 'fact' of the disease is contingent on particular political practices and processes, such as violent masculinities, the reliance on the male condom as a prevention strategy, massive youth unemployment, gender inequalities, poverty and the remnants of colonial-apartheid racial oppression. Mol's praxiographic approach offers a means of tracking these and other key political practices, showing how they contribute to making HIV and its subjects in ways unique to South Africa. It also allows me to draw attention to the possibilities and impediments in the lives of those affected by HIV, which existing policy formulations, set against the Mbeki–TAC conflict, fail to address adequately. By attending to specific practices, processes and relations through which HIV materialises as disease, we might simultaneously shed light on the self-serving or disadvantaging effects of certain materialisations. Made visible, these negative material effects are amenable to disruption, allowing a more generous, compassionate remaking of disease, one which guards against its latent potential to disadvantage and/or stigmatise affected individuals and populations. Crucially, if we accept that the ontology of disease is multiple and open-ended, then the possibilities for intervening to make disease differently are also multiple. In the context of HIV in South Africa, the question then becomes: how might we contribute to remaking the disease and, in so doing, help to reconfigure the contours of the epidemic?

Given that AIDS dissidence and political conflict have been defining features of the South African epidemic, one might hope that the idea of remaking HIV would hold some appeal. I suggest that HIV/AIDS can be remade in ways that move beyond the disabling disagreement over its presumed underlying cause and in ways responsive to the generative work of politics (including the disagreement itself) in shaping the disease and its subjects. HIV can also be reconstituted to work against the impulses of violence, stigma and fear that have dogged the South African epidemic. A first step to remaking HIV is to trace some of the practices and relations through which existing enactments of the disease have been produced. This requires denaturalising some of the dominant enactments of the disease, such as its symbolic association with stigmatised or vulnerable social groups, including men who have sex with men, drug users, sex workers and the rural poor. Throughout the book, I reflect on some of the possibilities for remaking HIV and offer some observations on how doing so might change the relational field of the South African epidemic. I conclude by appealing for an 'ontological politics' of disease (Mol, 1999, p. 74).[3] The concept of ontological politics presumes that realities – in the plural to denote multiplicity – are neither given nor fixed, but rather shaped within specific practices. The term 'politics', according to Mol, 'underlines this active mode, this process of shaping', drawing attention to the contingency and open-endedness of realities (1999, p. 75). Following Mol, the book takes ontological politics to include theories and methods of inquiry that address their own role (as part of an array of material-discursive practices) in producing particular enactments of the world and ruling out others. Such a politics challenges the self-evidence of the 'facts' of disease, revealing the political practices and processes through which disease and its facts are constituted. In this way, tracing the ontological politics of the disease HIV in South Africa has the potential to help remake disease in ways that transcend simple notions of 'fact' and their effects. Importantly, this approach does not deny the material existence of disease; indeed, it is centrally concerned with the question of materiality as it seeks to trace the practices through which disease is materialised.

In theorising HIV as an 'object in the making', this book also draws on scholarship from feminist science studies and the theoretical field often described as new materialisms[4] (Dolphijn and van der Tuin, 2012), notably Karen Barad's concept of agential realism. Responding to the 'discursive turn' in recent post-structuralist scholarship and its tendency to treat materiality as reducible to discourse, Barad offers a robust theorisation of the role of matter *and* discourse in the production of realities, without treating either as determining. In this respect, her approach provides a persuasive response to the problem of how to think matter and meaning together, avoiding the tendency either to neglect one of them or to instate a rigid ontological distinction between them. Agential realism pursues a kind of realism, but one that integrates the agency of objects (matter) in its realism rather than treating objects as the passive ground for agency. In other words, on this view, matter is neither inert nor totally determining, but an active participant in the making of realities (Barad, 2007). The term 'agential realism' is intended then to emphasise both human and non-human agency in generating what is taken to be 'real'.

To express the relationality of matter and discourse, Barad proposes the neologism *intra*-action. Where the more familiar term *inter*action refers to relations *between* separate, pre-existing entities, *intra*-action signifies that discourse and matter emerge through each other *within* phenomena: 'The relationship between the material and the discursive is one of mutual entailment. Neither is articulated/articulable in the absence of the other; matter and meaning are mutually articulated' (Barad, 2007, p. 152). If one accepts that matter and discourse are reciprocally constituted, it follow that an analysis of discourses of HIV/AIDS in post-apartheid South Africa necessarily entails an examination of the materiality of the disease. Moreover, since each intra-action produces a specific material-discursive configuration, an agential realist account requires scrutiny of the 'larger material arrangement (i.e. the full set of practices) that is a part of the phenomenon being investigated or produced' (Barad, 2007, p. 206). Therefore, undertaking an agential realist analysis of the South African political debate requires consideration of the role of the debate itself (and the kinds of action and inaction it produced) in making HIV/AIDS as disease. To illustrate this perhaps rather abstract point, my analysis addresses the material significance of the government's decision not to deliver ART, showing how it helped to constitute HIV as a fatal illness for affected individuals in poor and low-income communities, who rely on the public health care system (that is, the majority of those living with HIV in South Africa). For these HIV-positive individuals, I argue that the absence of ART in the public sector helped to cement, rather than break down, the link between HIV and AIDS: it effectively consigned them to death from AIDS. By contrast, for a small minority who had the financial means to access private sector treatment, HIV was transformed into a chronic, manageable illness. The point here is that the government's scepticism of Western science and its decision not to deliver biomedical treatment did not simply 'cause' deaths from AIDS; it contributed to materialising the disease – and those living with it or, indeed, dying from it – in ways that entrenched, rather than disrupted, socioeconomic inequalities. The analysis in Chapter 4 delineates these different, but mutually constituted, enactments of HIV, and it tracks how they emerge through the debate and the actions and policies it produced.

But how does one write an account that traces HIV in the making? Here, Marsha Rosengarten's (2009) monograph *HIV Interventions: Biomedicine and the Traffic between Information and Flesh* serves as a valuable guide. It offers a critical social analysis of HIV, illuminating the constitutive role of science in producing HIV as disease. In line with the theoretical approach adopted in this book, Rosengarten mobilises conceptual tools from feminist science studies (notably Barad's work) and social studies of medicine to present a compelling argument for the political and ethical import of understanding HIV as an emergent phenomenon, ontologically entangled with human bodies, medical technologies and disease concepts. Her work pursues a rethinking of 'the ontological nature of HIV as it is already inscribed with the affective contributions of science and social science/humanities' (Rosengarten, 2009, p. 108). The analysis that follows draws on insights first elaborated by Rosengarten about the making of HIV, and its deeply social character. While my account owes much to Rosengarten's analysis of the unfolding ontology of HIV, it contributes to the growing literature on 'disease in the making' by applying these insights to the case of HIV in South Africa, which is very different from the United Kingdom (UK) context where much of Rosengarten's analysis is set. This difference is important because if one understands disease as formed through political and social forces, then the socio-political context is not incidental to the ontology of disease, but rather imbricated in it. On this view, HIV in the UK is ontologically different from HIV in South Africa in that the two political-geographical contexts – with all the variable political and social practices they entail – produce the disease in qualitatively different forms, each with their own implications for affected individuals. The book traces some of the political forces that have contributed to the differential constitution of HIV in South Africa and, importantly, to the uniquely severe epidemic in that country.

Outline of the book: HIV/AIDS as politics

In pursuing the aim of the book to examine the role of politics in making the disease HIV in South Africa, I address four major questions:

1. How is HIV/AIDS materialised as disease in the TAC–government conflict under former president Thabo Mbeki?
2. How are these materialisations historically constituted?
3. How is the problem of HIV/AIDS articulated in the conflict and what role do particular problematisations play in shaping the disease in South Africa?
4. How do specific material enactments of HIV help to produce new selves for people living the disease?

These questions are explored through an in-depth qualitative analysis of a diverse set of empirical materials drawn from publicly available documents produced by Mbeki and his supporters, and members of TAC during the two terms of Mbeki's presidency and in the years immediately succeeding it (1999–2013). These include national HIV policy documents, public statements and press releases by TAC and the ANC executive, parliamentary debates, articles published in the respective newsletters of TAC and the government, legal proceedings, and TAC's health promotion literature (such as treatment literacy booklets and pamphlets). The texts analysed in this book correspond broadly with the focus of each substantive chapter:

1. contests over the science of HIV (Chapter 2);
2. HIV and poverty (Chapter 3);
3. disease as a politics of the human (Chapter 4).

The sample of empirical data analysed does not aim to be comprehensive, given the volume of government and activist material on HIV in South Africa published during Mbeki's presidency and in the years following it. It focuses largely on statements made by executive members of the TAC and the government. Of course, these cannot be taken as representative of the many different views circulating in government and civil society during the time of Mbeki's presidency. This caveat notwithstanding, the views of political elites warrant scrutiny, not least because they often have considerable influence on policy. In selecting the materials for analysis, I was guided not only by this awareness, and the three key themes identified above, but also by the book's overarching questions on the ways in which HIV is variously constituted in the debate, with very mixed and uneven effects for those living with the disease. The analysis followed an iterative, inductive logic: it involved cycles of reading, coding the texts for recurring themes, writing and reflection, drawing on concepts from STS and new materialist theory in particular.

I begin in the first chapter of the book by critically discussing the dominant scientific understanding of disease as fixed and given in nature, possessed of intrinsic biological attributes that determine its effects on the body. Drawing on the work of pioneering STS scholars Bruno Latour, Karen Barad and Annemarie Mol, the chapter challenges this view and its fundamental presumption that disease exists independently of, and anterior to, cultural and social forces. It ventures to explain how disease may be reconceptualised outside conventional ontological distinctions such as nature/culture and biology/society. As Mol has so compellingly argued in her ethnography of anaemia (1999) and later atherosclerosis (2002), disease is as much a socially and culturally constituted phenomenon as it is a natural or biological one. My reference to this body of critical social theory is in direct response to the polarisation of the South African HIV debate and the seemingly intractable challenge of reconciling Mbeki's AIDS dissident views with those of mainstream HIV science. Applying insights from Mol and the other STS scholars cited above, my project in this book is to recast HIV in South Africa to make visible the performative role of political, social and cultural practices – including the TAC–government conflict itself – in shaping the very materiality of the disease. Within a conventional realist model this materiality is ordinarily understood as developing 'naturally' and the substance of disease is taken to be the effect of a hypostatised biology. A key task of this book is to denaturalise this understanding and rethink the ontological status of disease without installing it as *either* fixed and given in nature *or* the effect of social-cultural processes, which appear resistant to change.

Although this theoretical approach offers a challenging start to the book as it asks readers to engage with seemingly abstract questions about the nature of matter, it allows me to introduce the key principles about the ontology of disease that underpin the book. I explore, for example, how distinctions often drawn between the biological (matter) and the social (discourse) preclude an understanding of disease as always already a biosocial, material-discursive phenomenon, that is, as much a product of social and discursive processes as it is the expression of a prematurely reified biology. This attempt to complicate the binaries so central to dominant understandings of disease is especially important in the context of the South African HIV debate because, as the following chapters show, both the TAC and the government relied on these and other binary distinctions in articulating their understanding of HIV/AIDS and in arguing for apparently divergent policy responses to the disease. The distinctions that binary oppositions make are not a problem in and of themselves but the work that they do to materialise phenomena can be problematic. For example, and as already noted, the government and TAC's reliance on binary oppositions was in no small measure an effect of a seemingly polarised debate, which I contend worked to materially shape HIV in South Africa. In pursuing this contention, the analysis works to confound the dualisms that dominated the debate and it offers an understanding of disease that moves beyond the enduring ontological distinctions presumed by these dualisms. Such an understanding offers a richer account of disease as at once natural *and* cultural, biological *and* social, scientific *and* political. The chapters that follow consider the implications of this reconceptualisation for the accounts of HIV mobilised in the TAC–government struggle.

Chapter 2 offers a close analysis of how the Mbeki government and the TAC responded to the accepted scientific model of HIV/AIDS. Contrary to existing research that presents TAC and the government as starkly divided on the issue of HIV, I argue that they shared certain concerns. Both parties were doing the 'boundary-work' of science (Gieryn, 1999, p. 405): tussling over the demarcation between science and non-science in order to establish the 'real' science of HIV. Significantly, both were calling for a science that faithfully represents the 'truth' about HIV. In doing so, they understood the disease to be a stable, pre-formed object, amenable to discovery by the right kind of science. Although this understanding might appear commonsensical, and thus unproblematic, it reduces disease to a static object that precedes human action, and thus displaces from view the ways in which both human and non-human actions shape the very substance of disease. I explore some of the pitfalls of this rendition of disease in the context of the South African HIV epidemic, before concluding with a discussion of how an approach that treats disease as always under construction might open up new ways of addressing the HIV epidemic in South Africa.

Introduction 17

The next chapter builds on this starting point to examine another important, yet often overlooked, commonality in TAC's and the government's conceptions of HIV/AIDS: their understanding of the relationship between AIDS and poverty. In an effort to resist what they saw as an exclusively biomedical response to HIV/AIDS in Africa, Mbeki and his supporters argued that AIDS is a disease of poverty and not simply the product of a viral infection. Concerned that Mbeki's position failed to recognise accepted HIV science and embraced an AIDS dissident stance, the TAC endorsed the orthodox scientific account of HIV/AIDS arguing that, although poverty contributes to the disease, HIV is an infection and its causes are viral. Both accounts, despite their differences, rely on a biological/social dualism: disease as either biological *or* social in origin. Crucially, the analysis illuminates how the debate's framing of HIV as either a biomedical or a social problem limited the effectiveness South Africa's treatment approach and thus, in a perverse twist, helped to entrench the epidemic. Challenging this dualistic understanding and its tendency to divide disease into ontologically discrete domains (which are then dealt with separately), I go on to argue for a reconceptualisation of HIV as a biosocial phenomenon, produced in the encounters of biological and social forces. Doing so invites a different formulation of the relations between HIV, poverty and racial inequalities, the latter two being important dimensions of socioeconomic difference in South Africa. Poverty and racial inequalities are typically understood as impacting on the spread of HIV, or as exacerbating the effects of the disease. This view treats poverty, inequalities and disease as separately determinate entities that interact with each other in linear ways to generate predictable effects. However, HIV/AIDS, poverty and racial inequalities can also be understood as imbricated or enfolded in each other such that they defy explanation using deterministic 'cause-and-effect' logic. It follows that poverty, racial inequalities and other so-called structural phenomena can no longer be regarded as ontologically distinct entities; rather they are part of the politics that makes disease and that contributes to variations in its distribution and effects.

Addressing the fourth question that guides this book, the chapter then takes up the issue of how those affected by HIV are differentially constituted by the government's and TAC's accounts of the relationship between AIDS and poverty. In doing so, it challenges the fairly commonplace belief that HIV pre-exists the individuals and populations in which it is found. This conception essentialises disease and those affected by it. Building on other critical social studies of disease,[5] the account offered here treats disease and the subject as constituted in relation to each other, and in relation to treatment, policy, scientific practices and public health measures. In this chapter, I show how the government's ideas about HIV-positive subjects and 'at-risk' communities co-constitute the disease, reproducing its association with poverty. While the government consistently construed poor people as especially vulnerable to HIV, the TAC depicted people with HIV in quite different ways before and after the delivery of HIV treatment in South Africa. Before ART was made available in the public health system, people living with HIV tend to figure in TAC's public discourse as casualties in two senses: casualties of the disease and of the government's poor policy decisions. By contrast, in the 'post-treatment era', affected individuals are routinely depicted in TAC's health promotion literature as agentive biological citizens, responsible for managing their health and staving off illness. In keeping with one of the aims of the book to critically analyse the binary oppositions mobilised in the debate, the analysis illuminates the binary logic invoked by biological citizenship and the normative ideals it instates. These ideals are exclusionary in that they allow only some subjects to qualify as citizens. Those who fail to conform to the norms of biological citizenship run the risk of being denied full citizenship and rendered non-citizens or failed citizens, with potentially very harmful effects. Through this analysis, I explore how the ascendancy of biological citizenship as a modern form of biopower risks creating a new group of marginal HIV-positive subjects in the South African context.

Chapter 4 builds on the deconstructive work of the previous two chapters to examine how the problematic of the human and its presumed opposite, the non-human, is deployed in the HIV debate to make HIV and its 'human' subjects. In particular, it extends the previous chapter's critique of biological citizenship by scrutinising the notion of the 'human' implicit in the ideals, practices and technologies of biological citizenship. This involves an analysis of TAC's health promotion literature in which HIV-positive subjects are addressed as agentive biological citizens, responsible for managing their health and staving off AIDS-related illness through acts of continual self-surveillance and self-care. Through morally inflected injunctions directed at autonomous, choosing subjects, discourses of biological citizenship valorise individual responsibility, agency and rationality, all attributes of the human imagined by liberal humanism. Perceived failure or inability to perform these attributes can operate to disqualify the poorest, most marginalised HIV-affected communities from full citizenship. Far from being immaterial, attributions of citizenship have significant implications for access to so-called universal human rights, including the right to life-saving treatment. They therefore bear directly on the bioethical issue of whether affected individuals live with HIV or die from AIDS. Crucially, extensions and denials of citizenship also shape the very substance of HIV/AIDS, helping to produce two qualitatively different ontologies of disease: a chronic manageable disease (HIV) for those who qualify as citizens, and a life-threatening debilitating one (AIDS) for those denied full citizenship and who therefore cannot access the rights and rewards attendant on it.

Together the analyses presented in this book offer a way of understanding and, thus, making disease differently. They are intended to reveal the complexity, multiplicity and open-endedness of the disease HIV, as well as to persuade the reader that disease, like all phenomena, is at once socially constructed and thoroughly real. *Politics in the Making of HIV/AIDS in South Africa* also attempts to challenge apparently self-evident facts about disease, exposing them as necessarily partial, constructed and open to change. Disease and its facts can always be otherwise. It is this open-endedness that yields both the promise and challenge of forging HIV differently. The book concludes by considering how an account such as this, which examines the role of politics in producing disease, might open up fruitful avenues for changing the HIV epidemic in South Africa and counteracting the harms often enfolded in it.

1
Disease in Theory and Practice

At the heart of the Treatment Action Campaign (TAC)–government debate was a conflict over the science of HIV. Concerned by the Mbeki government's reluctance to accept mainstream HIV science, the TAC directed its advocacy efforts towards educating affected communities about the science of HIV and anti-retroviral (ARV) treatment. Far from being confined to the era of Mbeki's presidency, these efforts are ongoing and underpin TAC's HIV treatment literacy programme in South Africa. An example of TAC's efforts in this regard can be found in a recent (2012) issue of their *Equal Treatment* magazine, which focuses on the science of HIV, presenting 'easy guides to HIV testing, prevention and ARV treatment' and a diagrammatic explanation of the 'HIV life cycle' (TAC authors, 2012, pp. 1, 16–17). This latter explanation of HIV science presents the starting point for this chapter. It offers a useful provocation to unearth some of the sedimented binary oppositions mobilised in the South African HIV debate (and in much contemporary work in the field of HIV). Refracting the science of HIV through the lens of feminist science studies, I argue that HIV, in its dynamic relations with individual (human) bodies reveals the tenuousness of traditional ontological distinctions between the human/non-human, subject/object and self/other. In search of theoretical tools that contest the self-evidency of these dualisms and make it possible to think disease outside their rigid confines, I then turn to scholarship in science studies, feminist theory and the emerging field of new materialisms. The chapter explains the theoretical import of this scholarship for the book's overarching concern to address the performative role of politics in materialising the disease HIV in South Africa.

HIV and the remaking of bodily boundaries

In virological terms, HIV is defined as a retrovirus: it is believed to make genetic code in the form of DNA (deoxyribonucleic acid) from its RNA (ribonucleic acid) and then integrate itself into the host cell's DNA. In this way, HIV 'is able to integrate itself into the biosynthetic mechanisms of the very agents that aim to seek it out and destroy it', namely the lymphocyte or CD4 cells[1] of the immune system (Kleine, 1994, p. 128). While this explanation is by now so well-established as to appear incontrovertible, I want to query some of the antinomies on which it relies and, in so doing, challenge the ontological status of HIV as a distinct non-human pathogen that 'infects' an otherwise pure human body. If we think through the following account of the 'HIV life cycle', as offered by the TAC in a recent issue of its treatment literacy magazine, it becomes clear that the virus, even as understood in conventional scientific terms, confounds the foundational dualisms on which HIV science itself relies:

HIV life cycle: How the virus multiplies inside our bodies

1. An HI-virus attaches to a CD4 cell by binding to the CD4 receptor on the surface of the cell.
2. The HI-virus empties its contents into the CD4 cell (infects the cell).
3. The HIV genetic code (RNA) is changed into DNA [...]
4. The HIV DNA is integrated into the infected cell's DNA [...]
5. When the infected cell is activated, the HIV DNA is copied into RNA (the raw material needed for a new HI-virus).
6. Sets of raw materials and proteins for a new HIV-virus come together near the surface of a cell [...and are] assembled into a functioning virus.
7. The virus pushes out of the infected cell [...] Thousands of new copies of HIV are made in each CD4 cell and these new viruses go on to infect other CD4 cells in our bodies. (TAC authors, 2012, pp. 16–17)

Drawing on the principles of immunology and virology, this account delineates seven apparently distinct steps in the trajectory of how HIV enters, infects and co-opts the body's immune system cells. Implicit in this scientific explanation of the HIV life cycle are three foundational assumptions that merit scrutiny. First, the virus and the CD4 cell (the human host) are posited as two distinct entities in which the virus infects an otherwise healthy human host cell. Here HIV is understood to radically alter the boundary of the body, compromising the immune system's ability to distinguish between its own protective cells and the destructive cells of the 'other' (the virus). As medical anthropologist Meira Weiss (1997, p. 464) explains, 'AIDS, more than any other disease, makes the immune system our body boundary. What crosses it alters the very self that the immune system defines and protects.' However, it is also possible to understand the virus as 'other', and the host as 'self' as ontologically entangled, emerging only in their relations. Indeed, as the process of viral gene transfer makes apparent (steps three to five in the HIV life cycle above), the boundaries of the virus and the host are collapsed, if indeed they were ever distinct. Extending Weiss's account, we can say then that HIV does not simply transgress the boundaries embodied by the immune system; in remaking the immune system and thus the body's perception of self and other, it *confounds* the self/other distinction and the idea of the boundary.

Second, the description of the virus and host (or 'infected' human cell) is presented as a faithful reflection of a pre-existing, observation-independent reality, which the apparatus of science has simply captured. Although this view of science has such widespread currency as to seem commonsensical, it neglects the possibility that the apparatus of science is productive of and embodied in what it otherwise presumes merely to observe. Figuring the virus, host and apparatus as separate, bounded entities involves a level of scientific abstraction, which, although analytically useful, suppresses evidence of their mutual constitution. In the words of Rosengarten, 'there is a certain abstracting out of what is involved in this mixing [the mixing of the virus, bodies and observational technologies] – on the part of science – in order to achieve a seemingly stable object *of* study *for* intervention' (2009, p. 29, original emphasis). This process of abstraction elides the performative role of the apparatus (the observational technologies and practices of science) in materialising the virus and the host.

The third foundational assumption that bears examination concerns the ontological boundaries between the 'human' host (as 'subject') and the 'non-human' virus (as 'object'). In the above account, these boundaries are presumed to be inherent and the apparatus of science is implicitly figured as an 'inscription device' that captures the interaction between them (Barad, 2008, p. 169). Yet, as already noted, the virus and host can also be understood as ontologically entangled, where '[t]o be entangled is not simply to be intertwined with another, as in the joining of separate entities, but to lack an independent, self-contained existence' (Barad, 2007, p. viiii). On this rethinking, the distinctions between virus and host are the effect of the scientific apparatus, rather than stable and foundational.

This alternative reading of the host–virus dynamic has implications for at least three enduring Cartesian dualisms, namely the human/non-human, subject/object and self/other. Through the process of viral gene transfer, the virus, usually seen as a non-human object, becomes entangled with the cellular structures of the human subject, collapsing the boundaries between human and non-human, subject and object. What emerges from the process of viral gene transfer disrupts conventional understandings of the 'human host' and 'non-human virus' as ontologically distinct, discrete entities. It illuminates the co-extensive relations of the host and the virus: the virus is at once human and non-human, as is the host, in its entanglement with the virus. Furthermore, human bodies always incorporate viruses and other micro-organisms and each relies on the other for their existence. Yet the biomedical understanding of HIV forever suppresses the possibility of the co-constitution of the 'human' body and 'non-human' micro-organisms. Invoking a fortress model of the human body, biomedicine depicts bodily boundaries as inviolable and, therefore, according to the logic of immunology, the task of the immune system is to protect these boundaries against incursion from exterior, non-human threats.

Critiques of science that draw on feminist and queer theory, have questioned the assumption that an absolute, oppositional distinction exists between the 'human self' and 'non-human other'. They have argued instead that these distinctions are always partial and provisional (see for example, Haraway, 1991; Martin, 1996). Relatedly, social studies of medicine, such as Catherine Waldby's (1996) critical analysis of HIV immunology, expose as a fantasy the notion of a pure human body when not under attack by supposedly hostile non-human forces. HIV, even as it has been understood in conventional realist science, undermines the traditional humanist notion of the 'human' as inherently different from the 'non-human'. In this respect, and to quote Waldby, the virus can be understood as, 'an ontological threat', disrupting the status of the human through the 'colonisation of human genetic identity with viral genetic identity' (Waldby, 1996, p. 1).

Perhaps most strikingly, the viral action of HIV undermines the distinction between 'self' and 'other' on which the body's immune system is believed to rely. Because the virus becomes integrated into the host's immune cells, the immune system can no longer distinguish between protective CD4 cells and destructive viral cells. The viral cells (as 'other') are understood to colonise the host cells ('self'), 'forcing the human cells to manufacture alien viral cells, forcing human identity to participate in its own infectious defeat' (Waldby, 1996, p. 1).[2] In agential realist terms, we might say that through the intra-actions of the host and the virus, the boundaries of the 'self' (the host) and the 'other' (the virus) become blurred with the effect that immune system response is compromised. The point here is the viral action of HIV reveals the fragility of the border between the self and the other. Yet because of immunology's reliance on an absolute self/other distinction in depicting the threat that HIV poses to the immune system, the reciprocal constitution of 'self' and 'other' is obscured.[3] In sum, I am arguing that, if we are willing to suspend our attachment to Cartesian dualisms and to a conventional biomedical conception of disease, HIV provides rich ground for querying the taken-for-granted distinctions between the human and non-human, the self and other, and the subject and object. Indeed, it seems that the matter of HIV invites a post-humanist, performative account that explores the mutual entanglement of these foundational dualisms.

To undertake the task of developing such an account in the context of HIV in South Africa, I employ theoretical concepts from science and technology studies (STS) and feminist science studies. In contrast to the objectivist realism of HIV science, I propose that the ontology of HIV (and that of disease, more generally) can be more productively understood as created through, rather than preceding, the encounters of humans and non-humans. Two points are key in this approach. First, that HIV, like all disease, is both socially constituted and thoroughly material. Second, that disease does not precede the interventions designed to treat it, but rather emerges through them. In other words, the very substance of disease varies in relation to the specific measures taken to address it.

Making disease in practice

As an entry point into thinking disease differently, I want to begin with the apparently straightforward question: What *is* disease? Although the question is deceptively simple and the answer may appear obvious, disease has been understood in quite different ways across different paradigms. Within the biomedical and social scientific literature, three distinct, but related conceptualisations of disease can be identified:

1. disease as a *biological object, given in nature*
2. disease as a *socially constructed phenomenon*
3. disease as *made in practice*.

The first approach, which corresponds with a medico-scientific understanding, conceives disease as a stable, unified object possessed of underlying attributes that determine its effects on individual human bodies. Medicine undertakes to discover these attributes, determine the associated causes of disease and intervene to counteract its effects. As should be clear from the critique of scientific realism offered in the previous section, the analysis conducted in this book does not assume disease is simply the outcome of a biologically self-evident pathogen acting on the body in predictable ways. However, the conventional view of disease (as a fixed object, the outlines, causes and effects of which can be articulated simply and in line with a general scientific consensus) is relevant insofar as it is iterated by both TAC and the government during the course of the HIV debate.

Although the medical scientific conception of disease holds considerable sway and informs epidemiology and public health responses, it is not without limitations. By assuming that the material/natural world pre-exists discourse and is stable and unchanging in its characteristics, medical science instates a kind of material determinism. The second approach above, which views disease as a socially constructed phenomenon, developed in response to this limitation of medical scientific accounts of disease. Corresponding broadly with social constructivism, it prioritises the role of social factors in the signification of disease (Singer and Baer, 2007). Yet, despite the varied and sophisticated arguments put forward in the constructivist literature, contemporary social theorists have critiqued its disproportionate attention to epistemological issues and its associated neglect of ontological concerns. In the spirit of this critique, Annemarie Mol (2002) raises two major criticisms of constructivist understandings of the relationship between disease and language. The first concerns weak constructivism, which holds that language shapes our understanding of disease, but not disease itself. According to this view, we have direct access to representations of disease (in language), but not to the 'external reality' of disease (Mol, 2002). As an effect of this presumed ontological gap, weak constructivism reproduces what Barad (2007, p. 133) describes as 'the representationalist belief in the power of words to mirror pre-existing phenomena'. By extension, representations of things are seen as more accessible than the things themselves. In this respect, a weak constructivist view sequesters matter from language and hence understates the agency of language in the production of matter. Mol's second criticism concerns strong constructivism, which overstates the agency of language, that is, the power to *make* reality in any way. Its ontology can be described as anti-materialist: it neglects the agency of matter by according language sole power to determine reality. Somewhat paradoxically, the approaches that fall under the rubric of social constructivism both minimise and overstate the agency of language; this is the variation in constructivist approaches that Mol's critique illuminates. In both cases, the agency of matter (and the materiality of disease) is neglected.

In an effort to circumvent the pitfalls of both versions of social constructivism – and their treatment of disease as a stable object that is discursively *represented* – Mol elaborates an approach that conceives disease as a contingent phenomenon that is *made* in practice. This marks a shift in focus from social constructivism's concern with discourse, to a concern with actions, that is, how disease is *done* (Mol and Law, 2004). To capture her interest in how disease is produced in practice, Mol coins the term 'praxiography' as an overarching label for her method. Central to praxiography is the notion of performativity. Mol and close collaborator John Law define performativity thus:

> Performativity [...] is another crucial complexity-relevant trope [...] knowing, the words of knowing, and texts do not describe a pre-existing world. They are rather a practice of handling, intervening in the world and thereby of enacting one of its versions – up to bringing it into being. (Mol and Law, 2002, p. 19)

On this view, practices of knowing are performative: they help to make realities. Applied to disease, we might say therefore that understandings of disease *matter* in that they co-create realities, constituting disease, its distribution and effects in significant ways.

Abandoning the familiar view of disease as a single, unified object opens it up to multiplicity. It allows consideration of disease as a 'texture of partially coherent and partially coordinated enactments' (Jensen and Winthereik, 2005, p. 266). And yet, despite evidence of the ontological multiplicity of disease, explicit contestation over what constitutes a particular disease is rare. In most cases, the different practices reassemble into an apparently stable, coherent object. The different enactments of disease seem to hold together effortlessly, but a lot of work must be done to move seamlessly from one enactment to the next: this work comprises coordinating moves, adjustments, shifts and side-steps that make the multiple enactments cohere (or coexist comfortably) and bridge differences between them (Mol, 2002; Mol and Law, 2004). In her praxiography of the vascular condition atherosclerosis, Mol (2002) traces the processes by which particular enactments are coordinated through the calibration of test outcomes. When contradictory enactments of atherosclerosis emerge in different locations of the hospital, these differences are resolved by allowing one enactment to prevail over others or translating one in terms of the other. For example, the medical diagnosis of atherosclerosis is divided into pathology and clinical domains, which bracket out how the disease is enacted. Ultimately, the clinical diagnosis of severe pain determines whether a patient will be operated on, even if the pathology report indicates that the blood vessel walls are not extremely swollen (the diagnostic criterion of pathology for atherosclerosis):

Under the microscope, atherosclerosis of the leg arteries may be a thick intima of the vessel wall. *In the organisation of the health care system*, however it is pain. Pain that follows from walking and that nags patients suffering from it enough to make them decide to visit a doctor and ask what can be done about it. (Mol, 2002, p. 48, original emphasis)

Although diverse enactments, such as those described above, need not entail contestation, in the case of the political debate in South Africa, the enactments of HIV/AIDS produced by the Mbeki administration, on the one hand, and by HIV activists, on the other, were seen as mutually incompatible. Partly as the effect of a polarised debate, HIV/AIDS was not cohering as 'an assemblage of situated enactments' (Jensen and Winthereik, 2005, p. 267). The coordinating, shifting moves that work to create the semblance of a unified object were fracturing and diverging. This disrupted the apparent unity and singularity of AIDS, stalling the national response while the state and civil society organisations fought to re-establish a coordinated, dominant enactment of HIV/AIDS. The analysis conducted in this book explores the multiple, distributed enactments of HIV that emerged during the TAC–government conflict. While these enactments are, in some ways, quite different, they are nonetheless mutually reinforcing. In their encounters, and because of both parties' implicit commitment to ontological singularity, they materialise HIV as a unified, stable disease, the 'truth' of which can be exposed through the 'right' scientific methods.

HIV/AIDS: a matter of concern

Because the South African debate treats HIV as a stable object that the right kind of science can apprehend, it strikes me as particularly amenable to an analysis through the lens of Bruno Latour's (2004) 'matters of fact'/'matters of concern' distinction. Writing in the wake of the attacks on the World Trade Center, Latour expresses concern that some critiques of scientific facts bear a discomforting similarity to the conspiracy theories that circulate after global events like the attack just mentioned. Such critique, he argues, is misguided because it emerges out of an 'excessive distrust of good matters of fact' (Latour, 2004, p. 227). To emphasise this point, Latour cites the explanation offered by French theorist, Jean Baudrillard for the September 11 attacks, namely that the towers of the World Trade Center effectively destroyed themselves, their structure supposedly weakened by the nihilism of capitalism. Social critique made in this vein tends to dismiss events such as the September 11 terrorist attacks as nothing more than illusions. In this sense, such critique can be seen as driven by a misguided quest to 'get *away* from facts' by 'fighting empiricism' rather than reinvigorating empiricism to bring us closer not merely to matters of fact, but to what Latour calls 'matters of concern' (Latour, 2004, p. 231, original emphasis). In expressing disquiet about certain interpretations of fact and calling for more nuanced forms of social critique, Latour observes that matters of fact 'are only very partial [...] and very polemical, very political renderings of matters of concern' (Latour, 2004, p. 232). According to this view, facts offer only shallow, partial accounts of phenomena, reducing them either to the status of immutable material objects or to that of social constructions, lacking any material substance.

A shift in analytic focus towards matters of concern has the potential to produce richer accounts of phenomena as simultaneously socially constructed and thoroughly material. More than this, addressing matters of concern entails an exploration of the many participants that must gather and hold together to call a 'thing' into being (Latour, 2004, p. 233). The term 'thing' has a specialist meaning in this formulation. It is used, following Heidegger, to refer to 'an object out there and in another sense, an *issue* very much *in* here' (Latour, 2004, p. 233, original emphasis). We might think of HIV as a 'thing' in keeping with Heidegger's formulation: a gathering of practices and relations that cannot be reduced to a simple 'matter of fact'. In its attention to the array of participants that must assemble to call a 'thing' into being, Latour's mode of enquiry seeks to add to reality instead of subtracting from it:

[W]hat is presented here is an entirely different attitude than the critical one, not a flight into the conditions of possibility of a given matter of fact, not the addition of something more human that the inhumane matters of fact would have missed but rather a multifarious inquiry launched with the tools of anthropology, philosophy, metaphysics, history, sociology to detect *how many participants* are gathered in a *thing* to make it exist and to maintain its existence. (Latour, 2004, p. 246, original emphasis)

Following Latour, one might say that realities (including the realities of HIV) are composed of matters of concern, webs of practices and relations that gather in 'things' to give them the appearance of singular, stable entities.

Latour's distinction between matters of fact and matters of concern is especially relevant to the concerns of this book. It offers a valuable conceptual lens through which to critique the TAC–government account of HIV, pointing out the inadequacies of treating HIV as a pre-formed object of science (or in Latour's terms, as a 'matter of fact'). Reading and remaking HIV as a 'matter of concern' involves problematising conventional 'facts' about the disease, revealing them as emergent and contingent, rather than self-evidently given. This reframing of disease enables an examination of the significant role of politics in making disease as it operates on the premise that 'conventions and values and social practices such as health policy and stigma make the disease as much as microbes do' (Fraser and Seear, 2011, p. 11). Furthermore, by querying the debate's rendering of HIV as a stable disease object (a 'matter of fact'), the analysis is able to reveal what has been lost in the political struggle over the so-called facts of HIV.

Agential realism and the intra-activity of disease

In pursuing the book's impetus to rethink the relationship between politics and the materiality of HIV in South Africa, I was also drawn to the work of feminist science studies scholar Karen Barad. Her influential book *Meeting the Universe Halfway: Quantum Physics and the Entanglement of Matter and Meaning* (2007) engages the question of matter without assuming either that it exists prior to discourse as a fact of nature or that it is largely a product of discourse and thus lacks any agency. Barad's starting point in developing what she calls her 'agential realist' approach is feminist scholarship. She engages directly with the history of feminist debate about the role of the body ('matter') in producing gender, aligning her work closely with feminist post-structuralist theories, notably Judith Butler's (1999) theory of gender performativity. As is well known, Butler's performativity contests the conventional view of gender as a marker of culture, inscribed on an already sexed body. Because this familiar view instates the sex/gender distinction in terms of the nature/culture binary, it reinforces a problematic conception of the body as an inert *tabula rasa* on which culture inscribes its mark in the form of gender. Butler's notion of performativity deconstructs the sex/gender binary by refiguring gender as an iterative effect of discourse, constituted through the repetition of discursive practices.

Despite acknowledging the important contribution of Butler's account in disrupting the sex/gender distinction, Barad is critical of the approach she takes to materiality, arguing that it fails to account adequately for exactly how discursive practices constitute material bodies and, more problematically, it reiterates the matter/discourse dualism by implicitly equating matter with passivity (Barad, 2003). Treating matter in this way neglects its active role in producing realities. In an effort to remedy this neglect, Barad is concerned to 'sharpen the theoretical tool of performativity' so that it might offer a robust account of the agency of matter in making and transforming realities (Barad, 2003, p. 803). Elaborating on Butler's formulation, she proposes a somewhat refigured concept of performativity that takes seriously the contributory work of both material and discursive practices in the process of materialisation. However, Barad does not confine herself to addressing the material-discursive tension and the related assumption that matter and discourse are ontologically distinct entities, indeed separate scholarly concerns. Agential realism goes further by exposing the mutual entailment of other traditional dualisms such as subject/object, human/non-human and nature/culture. It offers a way of rethinking their relations as entangled and co-constitutive. As Barad explains, agential realism is:

> an epistemological-ontological-ethical framework that provides an understanding of the role of the human *and* non-human, material *and* discursive, and natural *and* cultural factors in scientific and other social-material practices, thereby moving such considerations well beyond the well-worn debates that pit constructivism against realism, agency against structure, and idealism against materialism. (Barad, 2007, p. 26, original emphasis)

Agential realism's insistence on confounding traditional polar opposites is particularly apposite to this book, given its aim of querying the presumed polarisation of the HIV debate and drawing attention to some significant and worrisome commonalities in both Mbeki's and TAC's positions. More broadly, Barad's agential realist approach offers valuable tools for reconceiving the ontology of HIV and revealing its profoundly political character. To illustrate this rather abstract point, I offer the example of South Africa's social welfare policy as it pertains to people living with HIV. HIV-positive South Africans with a CD4 count of below 200 or 350 (depending on the measure) qualify for a disability grant (de Paoli *et al.*, 2010). Once on ARVs, an HIV-positive person's CD4 count rises and their improved health means they are no longer eligible for a grant and must resume work. When an HIV-positive person loses the grant, they are often unable to support themselves and meet basic needs, such as eating a nutritious diet to sustain the immune system. The stress associated with a loss of income and an inability to meet nutritional needs has negative implications for a person's ARV adherence and in turn for the disease progression as measured by their CD4 count.

Some of these issues were explored in a recent study of 217 HIV-positive individuals on ARVs in the Western Cape province of South Africa. The study, commissioned by Norwegian research foundation Fafo, showed that the threat of losing the grant prompted some people to adopt strategies to keep their CD4 count low to ensure continued access to the grant, without seriously compromising their health. These strategies included increasing alcohol consumption for a few days before a clinic appointment or skipping treatment (de Paoli *et al.*, 2010). One effect of skipping treatment (or, in medical terms, 'irregular ART adherence') is that it allows drug-resistant strains of the virus to develop. In agential realist terminology, one can usefully describe poverty, loss of income, individual risk calculus, irregular anti-retroviral therapy (ART) adherence, HIV and the ARVs themselves as intra-acting to produce drug-resistant forms of the virus. Furthermore, these phenomena, in their encounters with a narrowly conceived policy, can be said to produce illness among HIV-positive people in poor communities. Seen in this light, a policy originally designed to help HIV-positive people ends up contributing to the problem of AIDS-related illness by putting in place eligibility criteria that discourage treatment adherence and militate against improved health outcomes. It is possible to argue then that, in a perverse twist, the policy actually places an economic value on being sick. The title of a recent article published by Oxfam (the Oxford Committee for Famine Relief) highlights the conundrum that South Africa's disability policy has created. It asks: 'Income or Health? Can HIV Patients Have Both?' (Vasudev, 2008). Making a trade-off between improved health and poverty due to loss of the grant has serious implications, not only for the entrenchment of poverty in HIV-affected populations but also for the emergence of new drug-resistant strains of the virus.

On the basis of the above, we can read South Africa's disability policy as directly implicated in materialising HIV in damaging ways: the disability policy in its relations with poverty, illness, regulations on grant access, irregular ARV adherence, employment capacity and lowered CD4 counts acts to produce AIDS-related illness and drug resistance in some HIV-positive people. To treat these phenomena as discrete, anterior objects is to neglect the ways in which they are constituted through each other and through specific practices. In particular, it is worth emphasising how the mutating virus challenges the conventional view that it is an isolatable entity with inherent attributes. As this example makes clear, the virus is formed differently in specific encounters – or intra-actions – with bodies, drugs, policy, individual risk calculus and so on. Therefore, the ontology of the virus is contingent on its relations with other phenomena (themselves multiply co-constituted). From an agential realist perspective, the virus can be usefully understood as having an intra-active history from which its ontology cannot be extricated.

Conclusion

In developing this book's theoretical approach, I have been guided by a desire to move beyond existing accounts of disease as a biologically self-evident, stable object, which precedes politics. According to this familiar and influential view, the disease HIV has simply been exacerbated (but not materially altered) by government-led dissidence and poor policy in South Africa. This book draws on new materialist theories to challenge this conception of disease, proposing instead that disease – like all phenomena – is continually formed and changed in political practices and processes. Together, the theoretical concepts discussed here enable an account of the performativity of politics (including the TAC–government conflict) in making HIV. They allow me to analyse, and thus, remake, HIV as a 'matter of concern' (Latour, 2004): both as materially real, and as the effect of social, historical and political forces. Here I draw too on Barad's (2007) notion of the 'phenomenon', the primary ontological unit in her agential realist approach. Akin to Latour's 'matters of concern', phenomena are the 'result of intra-actions of material-discursive practices' and as such they are constantly (re)made in their intra-actions with other phenomena (Barad, 2007, p. 389). Since each intra-action produces a specific material-discursive configuration, an analysis that foregrounds intra-activity demands attention to the 'larger material arrangement (i.e., the full set of practices) that is part of the phenomenon being investigated or produced' (Barad, 2007, p. 390). Barad's interest in the 'larger material arrangement' articulates with Mol's (2002) concern to map the practices through which a phenomenon, such as disease, hangs together. One might say that all three scholars refigure realism: they appeal to a kind of renewed empiricism that engages the complexity of reality as a dynamic assemblage of material-discursive practices. Indeed, Latour (2004, p. 232) characterises his approach as 'the second empiricism' to distinguish it from conventional scientific forms of empiricism, which he argues reduce objects to simple matters of fact.

The approaches that Barad, Latour and Mol critique proceed from the persistent assumption of an ontological distinction between nature and culture (and, by extension, materiality and meaning). Furthermore, they tend to privilege meaning over matter and accord discourse the sole power to determine reality. In refiguring realism, these scholars are calling, not for a return to a modernist conception of reality as self-evidently given, but for an account of reality that conceives of the material and the discursive together. Their approaches incorporate the agency of matter into an exploration of how the world comes into being. Matter is understood neither as inert and passive, nor as totally determining, but as actively contributing to the making of realities. In this respect the theoretical trajectories that Barad, Latour and Mol pursue are consonant with what some scholars have called 'critical materialism' (Coole and Frost, 2010, p. 27), which draws on the insights of the social constructivist tradition but also takes seriously the materiality of the world. Following Barad, Latour and Mol's reformulation of realism, this book treats (and thus remakes) HIV as a matter of concern: a material-political-social phenomenon that is iteratively made in daily practices and is amenable to change.

To sum up then, I employ Mol's praxiography, Barad's agential realism and what I call Latour's 'renewed realism' towards three objectives:

1. to recast the history of HIV in South Africa, making visible the important role of the social and the political in making disease;
2. to critique the overarching common-sense realism of the TAC–government debate, revealing how it enacts HIV as a pre-existing object possessed of intrinsic attributes (a matter of fact); and

3. to rethink, and thus remake, HIV as an emergent, composite phenomenon that is both socially constructed and thoroughly material (a matter of concern).

In terms of the structure of the analysis, the first two objectives set up the terrain for the third in that (re)reading the history of HIV through the lens of agential realism and identifying the limitations of a common-sense realist account of disease, prompts the question: how else might disease, in both its materiality and its 'constructedness' be conceived? This is where the renewed realist approaches discussed above prove particularly apposite as they offer a way of thinking the material and the social together: they invite an account of disease as always already socially constructed *and* entirely material.

2
Contesting Science, Making Disease

Disease, as noted in the previous chapters, does not precede politics, but rather emerges in relation to it. It is a site of, and is forged through, ongoing negotiation. Or, as Fraser and Seear (2011, p. 142) observe in a sympathetic context – that of hepatitis C – disease is 'a site of dealing and dispute in its ontology'. This chapter maps some key disputes over the science of HIV that took place in South Africa under Mbeki and tracks how these helped to differentially materialise HIV as disease. It compares how the Mbeki government and the Treatment Action Campaign (TAC) responded to the dominant scientific model of HIV/AIDS and, in particular, how the 'problem of HIV' was constituted through their responses. In doing so, the chapter advances the broader objective of the book to trace the performative role of politics, including contests over science, in producing specific, sometimes harmful, ontologies of HIV in South Africa. Tracing the political processes through which HIV has been constituted is important because, when these processes change, so too does the substance of the disease. In other words, far from being irrelevant to disease and its effects, the workings of politics have the potential to dramatically alter the very materiality of HIV in South Africa and in turn, the contours of the epidemic and the lives of those affected by it.

I begin by examining Mbeki's critique of HIV science, in particular his use of the metaphor of racism as disease to challenge the scientised rationality of medicine. In mounting this critique, Mbeki argued that one of the biggest problems facing post-apartheid South Africa is the 'disease of racism' and not the disease of HIV/AIDS (as many public health practitioners and scholars claim). He further claimed that epidemiological explanations of 'African AIDS' reiterate racist stereotypes about African sexual conduct. In the process, Mbeki construes orthodox HIV science as 'bad' science. The government's critique of mainstream HIV science can therefore be understood as part of an appeal for 'good' science on HIV – that is, science capable of exposing the 'truth' of HIV in Africa. Implicit here is an assumption that good science will reveal the HIV epidemic in Africa as having nothing to do with 'African sexual difference'. Yet, as I show in this chapter, the implicit distinction drawn between 'good' and 'bad' science leaves intact the authority of positivist science. It enacts 'good' science in the realist tradition as having the capacity to uncover and faithfully record a transparently given nature – in this case, what are presumed to be the essential characteristics (the underlying reality) of HIV in Africa.

In the second part of the chapter, I turn to the government's supposed antithesis in the HIV debate, the TAC, drawing attention to an important (and worrisome) similarity in their approaches. In response to the government's expressed wariness of mainstream HIV science, TAC members sought to re-establish the scientific orthodoxy on HIV. Contrary to the presumed polarisation of TAC's and the government's positions, TAC also asserted the 'truth' about HIV as something that could be faithfully captured by science. Through their appeals to the 'truth' and 'reality' of HIV/AIDS, both parties in the debate enact the disease as a 'matter of fact' (Latour, 2004): a stable, naturally given object that pre-exists its encounters with science. Thus, to some extent, and despite their differences, the government and the TAC were collaborators in jointly producing this particular rendition of disease. Many implications follow from both parties' narrow emphasis on the 'facts' of disease but perhaps the most important is what it displaces from view. By insisting that HIV is a singular object whose underlying reality can be uncovered, the debate brackets out how practices (including the debate itself) make the disease: at every moment, the debate and the kinds of activity/inactivity it produces shape the epidemic – even as the epidemic is treated as anterior to the debate.

Challenging scientific orthodoxy: HIV and the disease of racism

In a parliamentary questions and replies session in October 2004, a member of the opposition Democratic Alliance (DA), Ryan Coetzee submitted a question about the role of rape and sexual violence in the spread of HIV: 'Does pervasive rape in South Africa and the prevailing sexual practices and attitudes of some men towards women not account, in large part, for the spread of HIV in the country?' (Parliament of the

Republic of South Africa, 2004). The question was prompted by a contemporaneous letter in the African National Congress (ANC) newsletter in which President Mbeki rejected a claim made by a South African journalist that 'rape is pervasive in Africa' (Mbeki, 2004b). He contended that the claim implied that 'African traditions, indigenous religions and culture prescribe and institutionalise rape', making 'every African man a potential rapist' (Mbeki, 2004b). Coetzee's question sparked a heated debate in Parliament, one that is worth quoting at some length because of its centrality to the dispute over HIV. Two representations of the problem of HIV dominated the debate: one in which HIV is bound up with the problem of gender-based violence and the other in which it is subordinate to the problem of racism. As the following extended excerpt shows, Mbeki resolutely refused to consider the representation of the problem as proposed by Coetzee:

[Paragraph 3] The PRESIDENT OF THE REPUBLIC: [...] I will only address the central issue raised in the letter in the *ANC Today*, and that matter is the issue of racism. Contrary to this, the hon[ourable] member wants us to discuss what he describes as 'pervasive rape' in South Africa, the prevailing sexual practices and the attitudes of some men towards women, asking whether these do not account, in large part, to [sic] the spread of HIV in the country.

[...]

[11] Whatever the circumstances and regardless of the regularity of Catholic incantations about playing the race card, I for my part will not keep quiet while others whose minds have been corrupted by the *disease of racism* accuse us, the black people of South Africa, of Africa and the world, as being, by virtue of our African-ness and skin colour, lazy, liars, foul-smelling, diseased, corrupt, violent, amoral, sexually depraved, animalistic, savage and rapist.

[...]

[16] Mr R COETZEE: [...] Mr President, this question is not about racism, it's about HIV/AIDS. And what you said in the *ANC Today* is that Kathleen Cravero, who's the Deputy Executive Director of UNAIDS [Joint UN Programme on HIV/AIDS], and Shaleen Smith [a South African journalist], are racist and harbour a stereotype of black Africans as, I quote: 'barbaric savages', because they suggested that the pervasiveness of rape accounts in part for the spread of HIV in our country.

[17] Now, Mr President, the fact is that rape is pervasive in our country and there is a lot of evidence that proves that. So in light of this fact and in light of the remarks that you made in the *ANC Today*, do you not agree that your comments did damage to the cause of gender equality in South Africa and to the fight against rape in our country, and that they cause harm to the fight against HIV?

[…]

[18] The PRESIDENT OF THE REPUBLIC: Madam Speaker, clearly the hon[ourable] member is not listening to what I'm saying. And I'm saying that the *ANC Today* discussed the question of racism, and I'm going to continue discussing the question of racism.

[…]

[41] Mr L W GREYLING [member of the opposition Independent Democrats (ID)]: Madam Speaker, I thank the hon[ourable] President for the reply. The ID has heard your comments on racism and we agree with you that it needs to be fought in this country and that it is a scourge that needs to be eradicated. But we want to restrict ourselves to the question of HIV/Aids [sic], because it is an issue that is important to us, in fact important to me because I've lost to Aids 10 people close to me.

[…]

[44] The PRESIDENT OF THE REPUBLIC: […] I have said that the government will continue with this programme on this matter of HIV and Aids, and I've got nothing more to add to that. We will continue to do as I have indicated.

[45] I have said before, and I want to repeat it, that I was discussing the question of racism and I am not going to be diverted to other issues simply because some members believe that the issue of racism is a minor question. It isn't a minor question, and we'll continue to discuss it. (Parliament of the Republic of South Africa, 2004, emphasis added)

In this extract, the Member of Parliament (MP) from the DA, Coetzee, depicts the problems of gender inequalities and violent masculinities as causally linked to HIV. In the process, he effectively quarantines the issue of racism, implying that it is irrelevant to a discussion of HIV/AIDS: 'Mr President, this question is not about racism, it's about HIV/AIDS' (Parliament of the Republic of South Africa, 2004, para. 16). Similarly,

Greyling, the MP from the ID, acknowledges the 'scourge' of racism but calls for MPs to 'restrict [themselves...] to the question of HIV/Aids [sic]' (Parliament of the Republic of South Africa, 2004, para. 41). Conversely, Mbeki prioritises race and quarantines gender by refusing to address the opposition's comments about masculinity and violence (and their link to HIV). Where he does address the opposition's question about rape, Mbeki euphemises 'pervasive rape' as 'prevailing sexual practices'. This euphemism normalises rape by failing to distinguish it from consensual sex (Parliament of the Republic of South Africa, 2004, para. 3).[1] Mbeki then goes on to attribute acts of gender-based violence to the 'attitudes of some men towards women', locating the problem with individual men, rather than with social forces that contribute to violence against women (Parliament of the Republic of South Africa, 2004, para. 3). At best, this depiction minimises the seriousness of the problem. At worst, it casts doubt on whether rape is a problem at all. Mbeki's refusal to acknowledge the ways in which the country's high rape rates are connected to HIV prevalence is particularly concerning given the feminisation of the South African epidemic and the 'nexus between violence, risky behaviour and reproductive health' (Abdool Karim and Abdool Karim, 2005, p. 258).

Furthermore, Mbeki's dismissal of the problem of masculinity and violence seems to be bound up with a general subordination of gender in his AIDS dissident discourse. As Marais (2005, p. 15) notes in his analysis of Mbeki's statements on the role of rape in the spread of HIV:

> There's a hint here of one of the overlooked hallmarks of South African 'denialism' – the overbearing male-ness of a discourse that is typically silent about gender injustices and inequality, and their role in the epidemic. At its core, this is a discourse by men about men, with women a shadowed presence here.

In this case, Mbeki is not merely silent about the role of gender in the epidemic; rather he explicitly quarantines gender and addresses instead the question of race, arguing that he is 'not going to be diverted to other issues simply because some members believe that the issue of racism is a minor question'. Refusing to address any further questions on HIV, he concludes: 'It [racism] isn't a minor question, and we'll continue to discuss it' (Parliament of the Republic of South Africa, 2004, para. 45).

Although it is easy to criticise Mbeki's dismissal of the ways in which HIV prevalence and violence against women are connected in South Africa, the opposition MPs' attempt to bracket out the problem of HIV from racism is no less problematic. It is difficult to escape the conclusion that the debate as a whole oversimplifies the entanglement of these social problems. In their effort to prioritise one social problem or set of problems over another ('racism' or 'HIV and rape'), both Mbeki and the opposition neglect the way all three problems help to produce each other. Instead, they posit linear, causal relationships between apparently independent problems (for example, 'high rape rates cause high HIV prevalence' or 'claims about "pervasive rape" in South Africa are a product of racist beliefs about the rapacious, violent sexuality of African men').

While it is common to explain complex social problems via linear cause–effect logic (where problems are treated as discrete entities and their putative causes and effects readily separated), these problems are more usefully understood as entangled, or, as Barad (2007) might put it, they emerge through the process of *intra-action*. The notion of intra-action illuminates, for example, how HIV/AIDS (an already co-constituted phenomenon) intra-acts with violent masculinities and the vestiges of racial oppression (themselves co-constituted) to help produce a disease epidemic that disproportionately affects young black women (Abdool Karim and Frolich, 2000, p. 5).[2] The ways in which gender, race and HIV are entwined is dramatically captured in an observation made by former Secretary-General of the United Nations (UN), Kofi Annan (2002): 'In Africa AIDS has a woman's face.' Equally, one could argue that the relics of racial oppression in South Africa intra-act with poverty, very high youth unemployment rates (Setiloane, 2012), a sense of emasculation among jobless young men (Boonzaier, 2005; Wood et al., 2007), violent masculinities and assumptions of male sexual entitlement to enable acts of sexual violence that place black women between the ages of 18 and 34 at increased risk of HIV. What I am seeking to highlight here is not only the connection between South Africa's history of racial oppression, gender-based violence and high HIV rates among young black women, but also the larger relational field which enables and cements this connection in South Africa. Doing so reveals that the phenomena of HIV, rape and racial oppression are constituted in their encounters with each other and with the effects of economic deprivation, gender inequities, massive youth unemployment, feelings of powerlessness among jobless young men and the (re)assertion of male dominance through violence (Boonzaier, 2005). In short, these phenomena are inextricably entangled. Treating them as separate social problems renders their relations invisible and so obscures the dynamic ways that HIV, the effects of youth unemployment, and racial and gender inequities enact each other to produce an epidemic that is unique to post-apartheid South Africa.

The articulation of these social problems as separate may, however, be politically expedient in that it allows policy-makers to reduce complex phenomena to apparently discrete problems, which can then be tackled with familiar strategies to generate linear, predictable effects. This view of social problems works to preserve the credibility of public policy as capable of achieving specified outcomes. However, by rejecting evidence of the relationality of social problems, it oversimplifies such problems and reduces the effectiveness of measures designed to solve them. Furthermore, insofar as the debate treats policy and its objects as distinct entities, it overlooks the role of policy in producing social problems, rather than simply responding to them.

As we have seen, Mbeki constructed the problem of HIV/AIDS as connected to the 'disease of racism' in post-apartheid South Africa (Parliament of the Republic of South Africa, 2004, para. 11). The use of the metaphor of disease here to describe racism bears detailed consideration. If we accept that meaning-making is material, then the question arises: what are the material implications of rendering racism as disease? Or to put this slightly differently, what work does this metaphorical language do to enact disease? Perhaps most obviously, to construct racism as disease is to mobilise an assemblage of disease associations such as contagion, infection, pathogens and quarantine. Although many diseases are, of course, not contagious, the metaphor invokes HIV in this context. Producing racism in these terms makes its threat more tangible and immediate. In Mbeki's discourse, the 'disease of racism' assumes the features of a public health crisis, deflecting attention away from the health crisis of HIV. Mbeki is appropriating the idea of disease and all it implies to shift focus from HIV to what he perceives as the more serious problem. As he emphatically puts it, in response to repeated questions from the opposition MPs about HIV:

> I have said before, and I want to repeat it, that I was discussing the question of racism and I am not going to be diverted to other issues simply because some members believe that the issue of racism is a minor question. It isn't a minor question, and we'll continue to discuss it. (Parliament of the Republic of South Africa, 2004, para. 45)

The metaphor of racism as disease also has a pertinent historical connection in the South African context. During the colonial and apartheid periods, public health and racism were mutually constituted concerns governing South Africa's health policy. For example, around 1901, when the bubonic plague began to spread in Cape Town, quarantine measures were implemented ostensibly to protect healthy (white) people against the risk of contagion. However, the forcible relocation of black Africans into native reserves as a 'quarantine measure' actually served the insidious goal of racial segregation (Swanson, 1977). It is noteworthy that this example was cited in a letter on HIV/AIDS co-written by Mbeki to the then President of the South African Medical Research Council, Professor William Makgoba:

> I would like to remind you of the story of the forced removals of Africans from District Six in Cape Town during the Year 1901 [...] Those who attributed the spread of the bubonic plague in Cape Town and elsewhere in the country in 1901 to the Africans, were similarly very certain about the correctness of their diagnosis. Once again, the fact of the matter was that this represented nothing but pure racism, a continuation of the process of the dehumanisation of the African people. (Ramatlhodi *et al.*, 2000, pp. 4–5)

The bubonic plague case exposes the racial biases of some public health measures designed to curb the spread of disease. It also shows how South Africa's racist policies helped produce the bubonic plague as a 'black African disease', even as they treated the symbolic association between black people and disease as pre-existing particular policy strategies. By creating the conditions for the disease to spread in the overcrowded native reserves, the colonial government's health policies helped to constitute the African subject as a disease vector.

The disease analogy is extended in Mbeki's construction of the problem of racism in that it is figured as a mental illness 'infecting' the minds of some South Africans: 'The psychological residue of apartheid has produced a psychosis among some of us such that, to this day, they do not believe that our non-racial democracy will survive and succeed' (Mbeki, 2004b). Figuring racism as a mental illness places it outside the bounds of 'normal' conduct. As with the disease metaphor more generally, this construction renders equivalent the struggle against one disease (HIV) and the struggle against another (racism), helping to emphasise the perceived threat that racism poses to South Africa's nascent democracy.

Implicit in the construction of racism as psychosis are the binaries rationality/irrationality and normality/abnormality, with racism associated with the devalued term in each pair. Extending the construction of racism as irrational, Mbeki argues that international organisations

Contesting Science, Making Disease 43

associated with the mainstream scientific community propagate 'hysterical estimates of the incidence of HIV in our country and sub-Saharan Africa' (Mbeki, 2000b). He continues: 'coupled with the earlier wild and insulting claims about the African and Haitian origins of HIV, [the estimates] powerfully reinforce these dangerous and firmly-entrenched prejudices' (Mbeki, 2000b). Describing estimates of HIV incidence as 'hysterical' challenges the scientised rationality of evidence-based medicine, implying that it is buttressed by irrational, racist assumptions about African sexual practices. Indeed, Mbeki is said to have contested the biomedical aetiology of HIV/AIDS because he associated it with racist accounts of HIV in Africa (Mbali, 2004; Wang, 2004). The reference to 'hysteria' here recalls Marais' point: it implies emotionality and irrationality, characteristics frequently conflated with the 'feminine' and, as such, devalued (Kirby, 2008). Mbeki's comment reinscribes this devaluation and, as with his refusal to consider the significance of gender in relation to the spread of HIV, it points more generally to a troubling treatment of gender in his statements on HIV.

By questioning the scientised rationality of medicine, Mbeki constructs orthodox science as 'bad' science for failing to adhere to the scientific principles of rationality, empiricism and objectivity, all characteristics routinely associated with the 'masculine'. By implication, he presumes that 'good' science is objective and impartial, producing verifiable facts about an apparently independent reality. This is the 'right' kind of science that the Mbeki government argues will help it develop 'targeted responses to the specifically African incidence of HIV-AIDS [sic]' (Mbeki, 2000c, p. 3). So Mbeki's criticisms of orthodox HIV science are made in the context of an appeal for 'good' science. It appears then that Mbeki does not reject the tenets of positivist science outright (as some scholars have implied he does by depicting his approach as 'pseudo-science').[3] Instead he seems to say, let us have the right science that will give us an accurate picture of HIV in Africa. Implicit here is the assumption that good science will reveal the 'truth' of HIV as having nothing to do with 'African sexual difference'. That is, the 'truth' will be free of the kind of racist, moralistic judgements that ascribe the severity of the epidemic in Africa to the supposedly deviant sexual conduct of black Africans. It is easy to see the appeal of this alternative notion of the 'truth' of HIV. However, in pursuing it and refusing to accept established scientific knowledge, the Mbeki government prevented a certain kind of action on HIV, namely the delivery of biomedical treatment. In this way, the government's approach contributed to making the epidemic and its effects more severe than they might otherwise have been.

It is worth noting at this point that the government's claims about scientific racism and its implied critique of scientised rationality find some parallels in the large critical literature on science. Many social studies of science challenge the deeply entrenched view that science produces objective truths about an independent reality (for example Edge, 1995). Meanwhile, feminist analyses of science expose the political investments of scientific epistemologies, including the ways in which science tends to serve masculinist agendas.[4] For example, Emily Martin's (1996) pioneering analysis of scientific accounts of human conception reveals the ways in which they rely upon and (re)inscribe traditional gender roles. She exposes the scientific language of biology as always already gendered, illuminating the ways in which women's bodies are subject to discriminatory scientific claims. Studies such as Martin's help to debunk the myth that categories such as gender and race are 'outside' the domain of science and that science is therefore neutral. They show instead that these categories are produced by science and are routinely used to naturalise social inequalities. Feminist science studies help to deconstruct gendered metaphors of science such as 'the traditional naming of the scientific mind as "masculine"' (Keller, 1995, p. 82), and they illuminate the relationship between objectivity (as an ideal of science) and domination.

Within the social studies of science literature, sociologist Steven Epstein's (1996) history of HIV/AIDS is particularly relevant to the Mbeki government's critique of the orthodox HIV science. Epstein challenges the myth of objective, rational science by demonstrating how biomedical expertise emerges out of political struggles. He chronicles the controversy over the causation of HIV/AIDS, tracing how established 'facts' were once the site of uncertainty and conflict. Through a careful tracking of how science is done, Epstein, 'lay[s] bare the intricate web of scientific argument, empirical data, and politics that has framed this controversy' (Bayer, 1997, p. 320). This kind of critical analysis reveals that, despite claims to objectivity, science is inextricably bound up with (and embodies) political struggles and disputes.

Where the Mbeki government's critique of science differs from the social studies of science discussed above is in its failure to problematise the status of scientific knowledge and expertise per se. Indeed, one could connect Western scientific rationality and the Enlightenment to the colonial reflex. Yet, Mbeki does not make this connection, which is rather paradoxical given his attempts to debunk colonial myths about Africa and his promotion of an African Renaissance agenda. Instead, in one of the most well-known AIDS dissident texts circulated during

Mbeki's presidency, Mbeki and his supporters reinforce the dominance of common-sense realism and scientised rationality by implying that the right science will reveal the 'truth' about HIV:

> It [a lengthy monograph explaining the Mbeki government's AIDS dissidence] recognises the *reality* that there are many people and institutions across the world that have a vested interest in the propagation of the HIV/AIDS thesis, because they have too much to lose if any important element of this thesis is proved to be *false* [...] It accepts that these have to be exposed to the *truth*, in the conviction that their consciences will enable them to side with the *truth* against the *untruth*, provided that they are informed of the *truth*. (Anonymous, 2002, preface, emphasis added)

This extract is excerpted from a lengthy essay titled 'Castro Hlongwane, Caravans, Cats, Geese, Foot and Mouth and Statistics: HIV/AIDS and the Struggle for the Humanisation of the African'.[5] The then chief electoral officer Peter Mokaba (now deceased) is believed to have written the monograph with assistance from Mbeki, although Mbeki did not openly endorse it (Shisana and Simbayi, 2002). However, as Wang notes, 'its rhetoric was so familiar that some speculated it was either written by himself [Mbeki] or by an assigned ghost writer' (Wang, 2004, p. 16). In the extract above, the appeals to 'truth' and 'reality' reproduce the 'positivistic image of science as an abstract, timeless search for irrefutable facts' (Edge, 1995, p. 18). So although the Mbeki government's AIDS dissidence exposes the orthodox scientific explanation for HIV/AIDS as political, it leaves the epistemology of positivist science unchallenged.[6] As a struggle against African oppression and the imperialism of Western science, it seems that Mbeki's AIDS dissidence collapsed into a form of internalised oppression, one that was ultimately self-defeating as it not only reinforced the dominance of positivist (Western) science but also impeded the delivery of anti-retroviral therapy (ART).

In his critique of scientific racism, Mbeki's invocation of the 'disease of racism' also highlights the performative dimension of metaphor. As I have argued, the mobilisation of the racism-as-disease metaphor does not merely represent racism as disease; it performatively constitutes it as such. In so doing, it makes the threat of racism more tangible and immediate. Indeed, it is possible to argue that, in Mbeki's account, racism assumes the features of a public health crisis, deflecting attention and resources away from the health crisis of HIV. The issue of resource allocation is a particularly important one as it bears directly on the availability and adequacy of national HIV prevention and treatment programmes. Not surprisingly, this issue attracted much attention under Mbeki with public health practitioners and opposition leaders criticising his government's HIV budget as being insufficient to address South Africa's rapidly growing epidemic (Hartley, 2001). On this basis, it is possible to argue that the inadequacy of Mbeki's policy response meant that access to HIV screening, prevention and treatment failed to keep up with the growth of South Africa's epidemic. This, in turn, allowed HIV infection and mortality rates to increase, thus helping to produce a materially altered epidemic, one which was more severe and entrenched than it might otherwise have been. Relatedly, Mbeki's refusal to concede the connections between HIV, violent masculinities and the feminisation of the South African epidemic arguably helped to reinforce the gendering of the epidemic.

I briefly noted that the enactment of racism as disease is shaped by historical forces, most notably South Africa's colonial and apartheid-era public health policies. I turn now to a more detailed examination of the historical connections between Mbeki's AIDS dissidence and his critique of racist science, as part of his larger struggle against the 'disease of racism'.

A genealogy of racist science

The connections between AIDS dissidence in South Africa and Mbeki's concerns about racist science can be traced to South Africa's colonial-apartheid history. Two aspects of this history are most relevant here:

1. the construction of the African body as a vehicle of disease in nineteenth- and twentieth-century medical discourses (Fassin, 2007; Youdé, 2007a);
2. the segregationist public health policies of the colonial-apartheid state.

In terms of the first aspect, the Mbeki government's resistance to the Western biomedical model of HIV is, as we have seen, bound up with what it saw as the racism implicit in Western representations of HIV in Africa. For Mbeki and his supporters, to concede the scientific orthodoxy on HIV would be to affirm racist stereotypes of Africans as sexually promiscuous disease vectors (Posel, 2005). Indeed, although accounts of HIV in Africa have shifted since HIV/AIDS was first named in July 1982 (AVERT, 2011), racialised constructions were not uncommon in epidemiological studies in the first wave of the epidemic (Treichler, 1999). Such research conflated the sexual practices of particular social groups (for example, Africans and gay men) with disease. In the case of the 'African HIV epidemic', the essence of its claim was that that Africans have sex in different ways and with more sexual partners than their Western counterparts, making them more vulnerable to HIV transmission. As Treichler explains:

> The reported [HIV] statistics from Central Africa were attributed to – among other things – 'quasi-homosexual transmission' [...] the practice of anal intercourse as a method of birth control, galloping prostitution and promiscuity (typically treated as identical) [...] multiple households/marriage [...] daily commerce with green monkeys and other suspect animals and various additional 'unfamiliar practices': in short, explanations based on the whole panoply of stereotyped 'differences' summed up by Paul Farmer as 'exotica'. (Treichler, 1999, p. 65)

In 1985, Africa became the focus of scientific research because of emerging evidence suggesting that HIV originated in West Central Africa. Claims about the 'African origins of HIV' contributed to increased media coverage in which the spread of the disease was depicted as a crisis decimating Africa (Treichler, 1999; Youdé, 2007a). This coverage, which was most intense in late 1986, attributed the spread of HIV/AIDS in Africa to the deviant sexual and cultural practices of African people that allegedly allowed HIV to be transmitted from African monkeys to human beings (Treichler, 1999). As public health scholar Susan Craddock (2004, pp. 3–4) observes, mainstream Western media accounts of HIV in Africa:

> tend toward unreflexive descriptions of cultural practices as causal factors. AIDS in these accounts exists because of [Africans'] entrenched fear and ignorance [of HIV prevention practices]. Such representations, damaging enough by themselves, in turn imbricate with and reproduce vestigial colonial images of Africans as ignorant, hypersexual and culturally backward.

Normative judgements about the presumed relationship between the sexual practices of Africans and the spread of disease were not confined to developed world discourses on HIV in Africa. Historically, South Africa's own public health campaigns had long operated on the premise that black Africans harbour disease and therefore constitute a threat to the health of the white population. In the early years of the twentieth century, when Louis Pasteur's germ theory gained ground, white South Africans began to use public health strategies as a justification for segregating the races as well as a means of enforcing white supremacy (Youdé, 2007a).[7] As noted in the previous section, the outbreak of the bubonic plague in 1900 enabled the white Nationalist government to use the provisions of the Public Health Act of 1883 as a justification for the development of 'Native locations'. Public health officials claimed that they were relocating black Africans to these designated areas as a quarantine measure (Swanson, 1977). The racial motivation for these separate indigenous areas is revealed by statistics showing that more white and coloured people were infected with the plague than black Africans (Swanson, 1977).[8] However, as Youdé notes:

> [by] placing black Africans into crowded 'Native locations' which lacked appropriate sanitary or health care infrastructures, colonial officials actually created the conditions for plague to spread among Africans – which only served to reinforce their ideas about the need to segregate the city's African population from Whites. (Youdé, 2007a, pp. 67–8)

Significantly, this was the first time in South Africa's history that segregation had been enforced in the form of native locations. These were to become a pillar of the apartheid state (Youdé, 2007a). Moreover, the use of public health measures to justify racial segregation was not confined to the outbreak of the bubonic plague. The spread of other infectious diseases, such as syphilis and tuberculosis in the late nineteenth and early twentieth century also prompted the use of discriminatory public health strategies directed at the black South African population. Notable among these was the 'deverminization' campaign conducted in Durban in the 1920s and 1930s where 50,000 black male workers were 'dipped' to prevent the spread of typhus (Marks and Anderson, 1984, cited in Youdé, 2007a). This colonial public health policy should not be understood simply as a response to the apparent concentration of typhus among the black population. My argument is that these public health practices rely on racial prejudices to enact the disease as a 'black African' disease, even as they treat the association of disease and 'African-ness' as pre-existing the public health practices themselves.

Fortunately, these manifestly racist policies are far removed from the current political order of South Africa's multicultural democracy but their vestiges clearly shape present-day politics and, in particular, the Mbeki government's understanding of HIV/AIDS (Fassin, 2007; Youdé, 2007b). HIV activist and South African judge Edwin Cameron makes the following point about the prominence of race in South African politics:

> A [...] history of racial oppression has forced South Africans, black and white, to confront their racial past. In national terms, we think racially – consciously, deliberately and obtrusively. We acknowledge the continuing presence of racial stereotypes and prejudices in too many areas of our nation's public and private life. (Cameron, 2005, p. 77)

When Mbeki took office in 1999, only five years after South Africa made the transition from an apartheid state to a democracy, the vestiges of decades of institutionalised racism shaped the tasks of reconciliation and democratic restructuring. This recent political transition, South Africa's history of racist public health policies and 'the politics of race, sex and death' that surrounds HIV in Africa (Cameron, 2005, p. 75), all facilitated Mbeki's construction of HIV as bound up with race. In contradistinction to some of the existing literature, I am not suggesting that Mbeki's AIDS dissidence was singularly motivated by a history of colonial powers using medical science to oppress indigenous Africans.[9] Or rather I do not see this account of HIV as a predictable outcome of oppressive, racist policies in South Africa's history. Instead, my aim is to excavate some of the historical forces that *co-constituted* the Mbeki government's AIDS dissidence, tracking how it emerged through a range of historical and contemporary discourses that enacted 'African-ness' as synonymous with disease, sexual deviance and racial inferiority.

Reading AIDS dissidence as produced by, and embodying, colonial-apartheid public health strategies and historical representations of African sexuality can help to explain the currency that AIDS dissidence held within a politics of African nationalism. This politics aims to 'change the terms of engagement between Africa and the West', giving Africa more political autonomy and economic power (Youdé, 2007b, p. 10). Locating the struggle against HIV within this pro-Africanist agenda could explain why Mbeki's AIDS dissidence endured for nine years (two terms of office), despite vocal opposition from within the ANC and from South African civil society more generally. It is also worth noting the possible importance of parliamentary politics to the persistence of an AIDS dissident government policy. South Africa's democracy was only four years old when Mbeki took office and one could argue that support for the ruling ANC was unshakeable, allowing the party to weather strong criticisms for its HIV policy and still maintain majority support.

Scholars such as Schneider and Fassin (2002), Butler (2005) and Fassin (2007) have argued that Mbeki's AIDS dissidence was partly an attempt to understand HIV in Africa as both a health and socioeconomic problem. They trace some of the antecedents of his position and are sympathetic to his attempts to reframe the problem of HIV in a way that engages the specificities of the epidemic in sub-Saharan Africa, in particular its connection to poverty. Like the above-mentioned scholars, I acknowledge the historical and social forces that shaped the Mbeki government's position but I support the widely held view that its public policy response to HIV was insufficient. And, although it is tempting to see TAC's response to the HIV epidemic as exemplary (and certainly their mobilisation for a national treatment programme was very effective), it also shaped the problem of HIV. In what follows, I consider how the government and TAC's responses, in the context of a polarised debate, have jointly helped to make HIV/AIDS.

Doing boundary-work: battling over the 'real' science of HIV

In critiquing the apparent racism and imperialism of mainstream HIV science, the government, in effect, depicted it as 'bad' science. In the following quotation, the government goes further, questioning whether the orthodox account of HIV is, in fact, 'scientific', arguing that it is 'highly tendentious' and that its evidence 'rest[s] on very tenuous grounds':

> The story we have told so far shows unequivocally that, at best, the 'scientific' story that is told about the 'HIV/AIDS pandemic' in our country, is highly tendentious.
>
> The more any open-minded person probes it [...] the more will this person find that what this 'science' states as incontrovertible truths throws up more questions than it answers [...] The 'scientific proofs' adduced to convince us about the various facets of the HIV/AIDS question rest on very tenuous grounds [...] The hypotheses about ourselves, that are presented as facts, rest on an age-old definition by others of what and who we are, as Africans. (Anonymous, 2002, Chapters 10 and 11)

The government's scepticism of the scientific orthodoxy on HIV constructs it as biased, empirically shaky and thus pseudo-scientific. Uncritical adherence to this supposedly pseudo-scientific account of HIV is judged a 'criminal betrayal' of African governments' responsibility to their people as it supposedly failed to address the unique contours of HIV in Africa (Mbeki, 2000c). By contrast, the 'real' science envisaged by the Mbeki government would reveal the 'truth' about HIV in Africa. This science, unlike 'racist' science, would be sensitive to the sociopolitical determinants of disease (such as poverty) and to the unique epidemiology of the epidemic in Africa.

In responding to the government's arguments about racist science, the TAC acknowledges the historical reasons for the government's wariness of science but is quick to caution against jettisoning its benefits out of mistrust:

> Some scientists during colonial times and apartheid misused science to claim that black people are inferior: we have a justified mistrust of the scientific community [...] But we cannot discard science and its benefits that are rightfully ours because of our mistrust. We would only disadvantage ourselves. We would lose science's benefits including knowledge, antiretroviral treatment, HIV-tests, medicines for TB [tuberculosis], electricity, flush toilets, comfortable clothes, radios and televisions. (Mthathi, 2006, editorial)

The claim that science has historically been misappropriated to serve racist ends performs an agential cut of some significance (Barad, 2007): it constructs racism as separate from the scientific apparatus.[10] The TAC therefore takes for granted the putative neutrality of science in this construction, with the effect that the explanatory power and authority of science remain intact.

TAC's editorial piece goes on to accuse the Mbeki government of misusing science to deny HIV-positive people the right to health care: 'We must not allow our own government to misuse legitimate questions about science to deny us our rights' (Mthathi, 2006, editorial). Here again the validity of science remains unchallenged (even as questions about the 'misuse' of science, and its effects, are seen as legitimate). It is merely corrupted by a government with ill-intent. Together these statements help to reinforce the cultural authority of Western science as the most reliable model for explaining what is assumed to be an independent, observable reality.

Consistent with its support of scientific orthodoxy, the TAC urges its members to '[j]oin our community activists in discovering the common sense of science' (Mthathi, 2006, p. 1). Depicting science as 'common sense' gives scientific knowledge the status of objective fact, foreclosing the constructedness and contingency of facts. In so doing, it performs another important agential cut (Barad, 2007): it naturalises science and its facts, placing them on the privileged side of nature. In other words, implicit in the notion of science as common sense is the belief that science produces objective truths about a transparently given nature, which is presumed to exist outside and independently of culture. This view of science is reinforced by Mthathi's (2006, p. 1) later assertion that 'science is not Western [...] we can all learn science and benefit from it'. I analyse this statement in more detail in the final section of this chapter, but at this point it is perhaps sufficient to query the claim that science is 'not Western', given that evidence-based science enacts Western Enlightenment values, par excellence. Constructing science as common sense also tends to efface the ways in which medical science enacts disciplinary power (Foucault, 1973). This is particularly relevant in the South African context because, as noted in the previous section, the African body was constructed as a vector of disease under the colonial-apartheid medical gaze (Butchart, 1998).

Despite their differing views on the science of HIV, both TAC and the Mbeki government draw a strict line between science and its presumed others, that is, those domains seen as outside science. In TAC's case, these take the form of quackery and pseudo-science, as the following quotation from its newsletter illustrates:

Pseudo-science can be deadly

Under former President Thabo Mbeki and Minister of Health Manto Tshabalala-Msimang the South African government was very slow to introduce ARVs [anti-retrovirals] in the public health system. Instead, they promoted false cures like the *quack* remedy Virodene and supported *charlatans* like Matthias Rath [a controversial doctor who claimed that nutritional supplements can cure HIV/AIDS]. Researchers estimate that this delay in making ARVs available within the public sector led to over 300,000 preventable deaths. (Low, 2009, p. 2, emphasis added)

By depicting the government's AIDS dissidence as 'pseudo-science', the TAC effectively dismisses it as having no epistemic value. TAC leaders contended, moreover, that pseudo-science propagates falsehoods ('false cures') that can be easily refuted through the methods of scientific rationality (Low, 2009, p. 2). TAC's emphasis on using science to distinguish between truth and falsehoods reveals that both TAC and the government endorse the traditional realism of positivist science. That is, they presume a one-to-one correspondence between science and reality. On this view, science reveals the truth of an independently existing reality. Where they differ is in their allegiances to the Western scientific model of HIV.

In challenging the government's AIDS dissidence, the TAC drew attention to its harmful effects, arguing that the government's 'delay [in delivering ART [...] led to over 300,000 preventable deaths' (Low, 2009, p. 2). Statements such as this point to the high stakes of the HIV debate: where real science is credited with saving lives, pseudo-science (in the form of AIDS dissidence) is blamed for causing 'preventable deaths' (Low, 2009, p. 2). The TAC also applauds science for producing apparently verifiable facts about HIV: 'Science enables us to know many things with confidence. With regard to HIV, we know that it causes AIDS, antiretrovirals save lives, condoms prevent infection and nutrition is important to maintain health' (Mthathi, 2006, p. 1). The scientific enterprise is depicted here as the locus of certainty and fact. Bound up with this depiction is positivist science's epistemology of progress: the idea that epistemic changes are part of a steady trajectory of scientific advancement. On this understanding, science advances towards the ultimate truth by observing and recording faithfully the inherent attributes of its objects (Barad, 2007). The objects themselves are presumed to be independently existing entities, part of a separate natural world. According to this view, science observes reality from the outside, and on the basis of these observations, it then discovers 'facts' about reality. These facts are taken as universal truths because they are believed to be the effect of a stable world beyond, and thus extrinsic to, the processes of observation and interpretation. For example, this is how TAC leader, Nathan Geffen explains the evidence that HIV causes AIDS: 'In scientific laboratories, HIV has been photographed numerous times. The picture on this page is an example. HIV has been photographed entering and exiting CD4 cells' (Geffen, 2006, p. 3). Geffen presents the enactment of HIV through the microscope as irrefutable proof of the independent existence of the virus. HIV is figured here as a pre-existing object, part of an 'unmediated Nature' that the apparatus of science can record (Kirby, 2011, p. 15). Although this conception might appear to be common sense, we can also understand the microscope as part of the apparatus that *makes* HIV. That is to say, and as I suggested in Chapter 1, the apparatus does not apprehend an anterior object, rather it contributes to its materialisation. According to Barad (2007, p. 195), the 'object of observation' (here HIV) is inseparable from the 'agencies of observation' (scientific apparatuses such as microscopes and photographs). So in agential realist terms, the microscopic enactment of HIV is produced through the *intra-action* of HIV (as object) and the microscope (as one of the agencies of observation).

Although this agential realist (re)reading offers a reconceptualisation of the ontology of HIV, it is not incongruent with the way that science has understood the nature of HIV. I am therefore not dismissing the existence of HIV as a destructive, material force. Rather, I am suggesting that the virus is more variable and dynamic than is usually recognised within scientific models that presume the existence of a stable, singular object that precedes human action. Crucially, this rethinking of the ontology of disease posits that HIV, like all phenomena, is constituted within human (and non-human) action and therefore the virus as it appears under the microscope 'is an approximation achieved through highly sophisticated but nevertheless selective [...] reiterative practices' (Rosengarten, 2009, p. 28). Because it is constituted differently in its encounters with different phenomena, HIV (like all phenomena) is ontologically multiple, continually changing and complex. It is also always with us, in the sense that we are in the world with HIV, not apart from it. Yet, to 'observe' HIV through the microscope is to materialise the virus for perception, that is, as part of a separate, independently existing reality. This realist view of the virus helps to create an apparently omniscient and detached observer as the subject. It presumes the subject exists separately from the rest of the world, including the virus. In contrast to this view, endorsed by the TAC, I am proposing that the subject, the virus and science emerge in their relations. In other words, they are intra-actively constituted. Importantly, the approach proposed here attends to the agency of matter – ARV drugs, the virus, the microscope and so on – in making realities. In contrast to the traditional realist approach iterated in the TAC–government debate, which holds matter as constant, so as to operate on it scientifically, medically and socially, I am interested in what happens when we free matter to act, to be contingent, to intra-act. What happens to disease then?

As we have seen, the HIV debate reproduced a view of science as neutral ('not racist'), rational, objective and evidence-based. Against this view, sociologists and philosophers of science have tracked how science is made (and changed) in iterative practices including contests over scientific authority. For example, sociologist Thomas Gieryn argues that science is 'nothing but a space [...] one that acquires authority precisely from and through episodic negotiations of its flexible and contextually contingent borders and territories' (1995, p. 405). Extending this spatial metaphor, we can see the different accounts of sciences that emerge through these negotiations as cultural maps. These maps secure the boundaries of science by defining its terrain against the non-sciences (amateur science, racist science and so on). What this suggests is that supposedly essential features of science might better be understood as contingent effects of boundary-work (Gieryn, 1995).[11]

In what follows I trace the good/bad sciences produced in the debate. Doing so involves recharting the terrain of the debate to highlight the points of continuity in the government and TAC's seemingly polarised positions. It could be an effect of the politics of the debate – and its presumed polarisation – that these connections were insufficiently explored. Indeed, media reports and scholarly analyses of the debate have helped (re)create the impression of a polarised debate. The account below is not intended to suggest that the government and TAC's sciences are either fixed or mutually exclusive. Rather, it charts the sciences that the conflict over HIV produced at that particular historical moment and, importantly, in the context of an apparently polarised debate. It should also be noted that the features of each enactment of science are not always consistent with each other.

According to the TAC, bad science is quackery and charlatanry. It produces falsehoods and endangers lives. Good science, by contrast, faithfully captures the 'truth' of its object and is therefore universally valid. It is the locus of certainty and fact. In short, for the TAC, biomedicine is good science. For the government, good science is African knowledge, not 'a simple superimposition of Western experience [and biomedical knowledge] on African reality' (Mbeki, 2000c). Such knowledge is sensitive to the local context, in this case to the specificities of the South African HIV epidemic. Good science, on the government's reading, is opposed to such bad sciences as imperialist science and racist science, which 'powerfully reinforce [...] dangerous and firmly-entrenched prejudices [about black African people]' (Mbeki, 2000b). By contrast, good science is equitable and just and does not discriminate on the basis of race (or any other marker of difference). According to the government, bad science is irrational in that it 'propagate[s] hysterical estimates of the incidence of HIV in our country and sub-Saharan Africa' (Mbeki, 2000b).

Given the tendency to depict the HIV debate as starkly split, what is perhaps most revealing about the sciences produced by the debate is the overlapping terrain of good science both parties share. The presumption of a polarised debate belies this shared ground. Both the TAC and the government enact good science as objective, evidence-based, capable of uncovering truth and thus producing verifiable facts. In this respect, both parties endorse and reproduce science in the positivist tradition. In the next section, I consider how their reliance on positivist science shapes the materiality of HIV in specific and sometimes counterproductive ways. As part of questioning the debate's apparent polarisation, it is worth considering the possibility that, had the TAC taken a less conventional, more critical approach to biomedicine, it might have allowed the government to concede some of TAC's arguments for treatment. Was the government painted into a corner such that it felt compelled to adhere to an indefensible position? Conversely, did the patent insufficiency of the government's position push TAC leaders to embrace biomedicine as the only available response? While there are, of course, no simple answers to these questions, the point here is that the presumed polarisation of the debate has precluded consideration of these, and no doubt other, pertinent questions. More importantly, as the next section reveals, the depiction of the debate as polarised has also materially shaped HIV in South Africa, limiting the available policy responses and thus impacting deleteriously on the distribution, course and effects of the epidemic.

Rendering HIV/AIDS a 'matter of fact'

As we have seen, several important points of continuity existed in the government and TAC's positions on HIV. Despite these continuities, the debate was framed in terms of a series of binary oppositions, a noteworthy one being science/politics. The distinction drawn between science and politics can be seen in the following statement by Mbeki, in which he responds to civil society's call for him to take an HIV test publicly:

> Let's stop politicising this question. Let's deal with the science of it. The panel said one of the things we have got to do is to determine when you do an HIV test what is the test testing. And those were the scientists: what is it measuring. So I go and do a test I'm confirming a particular paradigm. It doesn't help in addressing this health need. Our focus must be how do we improve the health of our people and that is what we are focused on. (Mbeki, 2001)

By framing his position as a non-partisan attempt to address the apparent lack of scientific consensus on the viral causation of AIDS, Mbeki draws a strict boundary between science and politics. His appeal to 'stop politicising the question [of HIV]' implies that if the science/politics boundary is crossed, the objectivity of science will be threatened, tainted by its contact with politics and the supposed lack of neutrality that goes with it. In contradistinction to his pursuit of the 'science [of HIV]', Mbeki characterises the call for him to have an HIV test a 'publicity stunt' in the sense that it promotes a particular epistemology (captured by the term *paradigm* in the above quotation) (Mbeki, 2001). It therefore goes against his quest for scientific neutrality. At first blush, this pro-science tack appears rather paradoxical, given Mbeki's critique of orthodox HIV science, but it was arguably an attempt to garner some credibility for a position that was widely criticised as non-scientific.

Although the Mbeki administration tended to frame science as capable of insulating itself from the effects of politics (and therefore, as potentially neutral), it did not consistently construct the boundaries between science and politics as impermeable. In a lengthy exposition of their stance, Mbeki and a member of the ANC executive, Peter Mokaba, observed that disease is both scientific and 'profoundly political' (Anonymous, 2002, preface). The boundaries between politics and science are here seen as relatively porous, but not completely permeable. This understanding of the connections between science and politics allows the strategic exploitation of the cachet of scientific expertise. The government is able to justify its policy decisions by their 'perceived grounding in authoritative and objective understandings of the facts as only science provides' (Gieryn, 1995, p. 435). Conversely, by acknowledging that disease is political, the Mbeki government is able to draw attention to the global inequities and colonial legacies that make Africa most susceptible to the HIV epidemic. Despite the political expedience of this move, the blurring of boundaries between science and politics still assumes that they are intrinsically separate, and therefore that scientific domains can be insulated from political ones.

Where the government sometimes acknowledged that science is shaped by politics, the TAC tended to construe science as thoroughly neutral and impartial:

> Many ask, whose science is it anyway? Why should we listen to a way of understanding the world imposed on us by the West? But science is not Western or mysterious: we can all learn science and benefit from it. (Mthathi, 2006, p. 1)

This statement by TAC's former chairperson depicts the practices and products of scientific inquiry as fairly distributed, and thus implies that science is benevolent. But if we scrutinise this claim, drawing on the example of HIV drug trials in developing countries, it becomes clear that it is empirically shaky. The success of off-shore HIV trials depends on the availability of experimental populations who, by virtue of poverty, food insecurity and other social disadvantages, are seen as vulnerable to HIV infection (Shah, 2006). Research subjects in these trials are typically impoverished people with limited access to health care facilities and little or no exposure to medication (Shah, 2006; Treichler, 1999). In the objectifying discourse of science, they are 'pharmacologically virgin' and so make ideal subjects for clinical trials (Treichler, 1999, p. 120). Indeed, as Rosengarten and Michael argue in relation to Pre-Exposure Prophylaxis (PrEP) drug trials for HIV, these off-shore trials do not simply rely on the availability of vulnerable, 'pharmacologically virgin' populations, they help to constitute this vulnerability. They produce a 'tragic quandary' in that they 'involve the very drugs unavailable or difficult to access for keeping people alive, with the knock-on effect of increasing vulnerability culturally (through, for example, undermining existing prevention practices) and materially (through increased viral resistance and drug side-effects)' (Rosengarten and Michael, 2009, p. 190).

If one recognises HIV vulnerability as partly a constitutive effect of some scientific trials, it becomes difficult to sustain the argument that science is intrinsically fair and can benefit everyone. However, Mthathi does go on to acknowledge that 'scientists in the West get much more research and training funding than developing world scientists' (Mthathi, 2006, p. 1). Developing world scientists may well be financially disadvantaged compared to their counterparts in wealthy developed countries. However, the subjects of clinical trials are almost certainly more disadvantaged than the scientists in the developing world, not least because they bear the burden of pharmaceutical drug trials but seldom enjoy the medical advances that they produce (Patton, 1990; Rosengarten and Michael, 2009). Indeed, it seems cruelly ironic that ART 'has been optimized for the richest 2% of those infected' (Grant et al., 2005, cited in Rosengarten and Michael, 2009, p. 192). This means that, for the remaining 98 per cent, two-thirds of whom are in sub-Saharan Africa (AVERT, 2008), ART has the potential to be only partially effective. In short, TAC's acknowledgement of the asymmetries in developed and developing world research funding neglects the more troubling asymmetries between rich and poor, healthy and sick that scientific drug trials help to (re)produce. As Rosengarten and Michael's analysis reveals, the design and outcomes of clinical trials for HIV drugs can be said to *cultivate* the research subjects' increased

Contesting Science, Making Disease 59

risk of contracting HIV. Crucially, their analysis disrupts the assumed distinction between science and politics, showing how science *'contains politics'* (Mol and Berg, 1998, p. 8, original emphasis): in the case of HIV, scientific practices tend to operate to benefit a small, wealthy minority, while exploiting and reproducing HIV vulnerabilities in developing world communities.

The science/politics binary articulates with another well-worn dualism mobilised in the HIV debate, namely biology/society. I argue that understanding HIV via this dualism enacts the disease as a matter of fact: a pre-formed, stable object possessed of putatively distinct biological and social dimensions. As noted in Chapter 1, facts offer partial, shallow accounts of phenomena (Latour, 2004). To trace the reductive effects of materialising HIV as a matter of fact within apparently separable biological/social domains, I consider an example from TAC's treatment plan. This plan draws a distinction between the biomedical and the social to argue that an ART programme should not comprise a 'purely medical response' but needs to be supported by strategies that address the 'social and development challenges' of HIV (TAC Science and Research Committee, 2001, pp. 11, 14). These strategies are described as 'non-health components' and include HIV literacy programmes and a basic income support grant (TAC Science and Research Committee, 2001, p. 14). As post-structuralist and deconstructive scholars have made clear, binaries routinely construct hierarchies (Bacchi, 2009; Derrida, 1982). In this case, the equation of social strategies with 'non-health components' points to the primacy of medical responses in TAC's model of disease. They are the default; social or 'non-health' measures merely support them. Understanding HIV in this way assumes that medical and social domains can be easily separated, an assumption that neglects the constitution of the disease as always already medico-social. It also prioritises treatment (as a largely 'medical' measure) over prevention ('social-behavioural' measures). The separation of treatment and prevention measures is not consistent with current thinking on the treatment–prevention nexus and the associated arguments for a 'treatment-as-prevention' approach (Montaner, 2011). Furthermore, treating HIV as a biologically given object (the 'target' of medicine) impoverishes understandings of the disease and the dynamic web of intra-actions in which it is made. Conceiving – and therefore materially producing – HIV as a biologically given object will not help to explain why, for example, HIV in sub-Saharan Africa is a mass heterosexual epidemic, yet in developed Western countries it remains largely confined to particular demographic groups. As Mbeki's critique of Western science makes clear, HIV is also deeply social and political: it is no coincidence that those who bear the burden of the epidemic in South Africa are poor, black and female, with almost one in three women aged 25 to 29 living with HIV (National Antenatal Sentinel HIV and Syphilis Prevalence Survey, 2008).

To draw these points together, the HIV debate made a series of agential cuts (Barad, 2007) between science and non-science, science and politics, and between the biomedical and the social. By constructing science as 'outside of politics', the debate excluded the possibility of thinking science and politics together. Yet the demarcation of politics as firmly outside the borders of science has a clear function in the context of the South African battle over HIV: it elevates science as the only model capable of uncovering the 'truth' about the disease. This view, in turn, helps to produce HIV as a pre-formed, stable disease or, in Latour's terms, as a matter of fact. Matters of fact, he argues, are 'only very partial [...] political renderings of matters of concern and only a subset of what could be called *states of affairs*' (Latour, 2004, p. 232, original emphasis). By insisting that HIV is a singular, stable object whose underlying reality ('truth') can be revealed, the debate brackets out how practices (including the debate itself) make the disease: at every moment, the debate and the kinds of activity/inactivity it produces shape the epidemic – even as the epidemic is treated as anterior to the debate. To illustrate this point, it is helpful to consider how the very terms of the debate impacted on the direction of HIV policy, and, indeed, the course of the epidemic in South Africa.

The framing of the HIV debate in polarised terms meant that, for political reasons, each party tended not to concede the legitimacy of the other's position. This led them to single out certain strategies for addressing HIV (such as prevention over treatment or vice versa), ruling out, at least for a time, the possibility of less polarised and therefore more effective responses to the epidemic; that is, responses attentive both to the complexities of HIV/AIDS and to the entanglement of prevention and treatment. For example, the Mbeki government constructed prevention and treatment as separate policy strategies, prioritising prevention measures over treatment:

> In the absence of a cure, our response to HIV and AIDS emphasizes the centrality of prevention. We are intensifying our programme to encourage especially young people to abstain from sex and those who are sexually active to be faithful to one partner. We are proactively marketing the free high quality male condoms and their distribution

has increased by 80% over the past six years. (Tshabalala-Msimang, 2004)

As this quotation suggests, the government's prevention model treats the spread of HIV as largely a social-behavioural problem – as opposed to a biomedical one. Given the criticisms of AIDS denialism levelled against the Mbeki government, it is worth noting that their behavioural approach is also part of the Western public health model, a model that the TAC itself would otherwise endorse in pursuing the orthodox biomedical approach to HIV. The intention here is not to imply that the behavioural model on its own is the best approach to HIV. Rather, it is to complicate the common criticism that Mbeki's approach was wholly illegitimate and indeed, diametrically opposed to the scientific orthodoxy on HIV. Such a criticism seems simplistic given that elements of Mbeki's approach correspond with the findings of critical epidemiological studies on HIV and indeed with the mainstream Western public health approach. The latter is, however, not without its problems, the most notable being its presumption that all that is needed to prevent HIV transmission is for 'rational' actors to change their behaviour (King, 1999). This leaves unexamined the ways in which a person's ability and volition to protect against HIV transmission is entangled with material-discursive practices, such as the reliance on male condoms as a prevention strategy, the practicalities of negotiating condom usage, calculations of sexual risk, and gendered discourses of sexuality and the silences surrounding these.

Moreover, implicit in the government's behavioural change approach to prevention is the belief in an inherent distinction between the biological and the social dimensions of disease. By reiterating this distinction, the government divides the complex phenomenon of HIV into two apparently discrete domains, which it assumes can be dealt with separately. This only elides evidence of the reciprocal constitution of the biological and the social (Barad, 2007): HIV is always already a biosocial phenomenon as it is produced in the encounters of biological and social forces. To analyse and treat HIV relative to these seemingly distinct categories is to impoverish our understanding of the disease and to diminish the effectiveness of our attempts to address it.

As regards TAC's response to addressing HIV, the polarisation of the debate and TAC's emphasis on science in the form of biomedicine may have pushed the organisation to embrace a policy that focused heavily on ART as the most worthwhile solution. Indeed, biomedicine's authority, combined with its inability to deliver on a vaccine or cure for HIV, has pushed the management of HIV globally towards an approach dominated by ARVs. Commenting on the shift to a treatment-as-prevention approach, Nguyen et al. (2011, p. 291) describe the increasing emphasis on HIV treatment as part of a 'striking remedicalization of our approach to the [...] epidemic'. This approach reduces disease to a medical 'object' that can be 'targeted' using pharmaceutical drugs and other biomedical technologies. In turn, the drugs are framed as *inter*acting with HIV to generate predictable effects, such as reducing viral load. In a departure from this familiar view and its presumption that objects exist independently of each other, I suggest that HIV, biomedical technologies and their so-called 'targets' can usefully be understood as existing only in their relations, or as Barad might put it, as *intra*-acting to produce each other. For example, ARVs intra-act with the body as their 'target' to produce not only a managed viral load but also a materially different embodied subject (Rosengarten, 2009). The subject is therefore formed, in part, through ARVs. Moreover, in their encounters with HIV and with social practices of drug adherence and consumption, ARVs help to create drug-resistant strains of HIV, thus re-forming the virus. One important benefit of this understanding is that it has the potential to enable the design of prevention and treatment measures that address the relationality and complexity of the problem of HIV. These measures might include the development of ARV drugs responsive to the variability of the virus; that is, the ways in which it is variously constituted in relation to the drugs themselves, as well as in relation to dosing regimes, drug side-effects, practices of drug adherence, drug absorption rates, the genetic characteristics of affected individuals, the presence of other sexually transmitted infections and the viral load test. Making drug design responsive to the variability (and relationality) of HIV would likely be more effective in addressing the disease – and thus in addressing other co-constituted problems such as viral mutations and drug resistance – than are existing measures, which treat HIV as a separate problem with clearly defined boundaries and determinate properties.

Furthermore, although it is common to understand HIV as a biomedical object (a simple 'matter of fact'), this conception effectively universalises the problem by constructing the epidemic in sub-Saharan Africa in the same terms as the epidemic in the developed world. This has helped to create a gap between international HIV policy recommendations and the specificities of local epidemics. As Campbell and Williams (1999, p. 136) put it, '[t]he language of HIV prevention has become the language of Western science and Western policy approaches, unmediated by an appreciation of the extent to which these are inappropriate for local conditions'. On this basis, it is possible to argue that the enactment of HIV as a fixed and stable object, amenable to medical treatment, has contributed to the occlusion of the unique ontologies of HIV in South Africa. It has thus precluded the design of more locally appropriate – and, therefore more effective – forms of prevention and treatment. For example, as the analysis in Chapter 3 reveals, HIV, in many cases, embodies and helps to reproduce poverty in South Africa. Yet the co-constitution of poverty and HIV has largely been ignored in the pursuit of a biomedical approach, which treats HIV infection as the result of individual conduct, presumed to be within the control of the rational, agentive subject. Consequently, biomedicine tends to prioritise individualistic behaviour change strategies, sometimes at the expense of those that address what are usually seen as the social dimensions of HIV. In the South African case, these so-called social dimensions include the association of HIV with poverty, socio-political marginalisation, crowded informal living conditions, limited access to sanitation facilities and a struggling public health system. Within the influential biomedical model, these social factors are typically seen as secondary, if not irrelevant, to disease aetiology and thus outside the ambit of medical intervention (Fee and Krieger, 1993).

The renewed emphasis on biomedical measures in the post-ART phase of the epidemic is also the effect of the heroic discourse of biomedicine which, despite its important contribution to managing HIV/AIDS, remains unable to provide two key medical solutions to disease: prevention (vaccine) and cure (Rosengarten, 2009). And yet the emergence of ART has helped reinforce the epistemological credibility of biomedical responses to HIV, diminishing the important critiques of science and biomedicine which figured prominently in the first wave of the epidemic and which revealed some of the limits of a biomedical approach (Mykhalovskiy and Rosengarten, 2009). Against the proliferation of biomedical responses to HIV, scholars such as Mykhalovskiy and Rosengarten (2009) have appealed for renewed critical social inquiry into HIV. Along with Rosengarten (2009), Fraser and Seear (2011) and others, I argue that agential realism offers a theoretical entry point for such critical scholarly engagement as it enables an account of disease, not as a naturally given scientific object but as an emergent social-material phenomenon, forged through (rather than preceding) our attempts to know it. By refiguring disease in this way, agential realism allows an analysis of HIV/AIDS as an 'object-in-the making', made and changed at the gathering of science, politics, racism,

African nationalism, sexuality, gender, AIDS dissidence and many other phenomena.

Conclusion

A key concern underpinning the Mbeki government's critique of HIV science was not the disease HIV, but the 'disease of racism' that has characterised much of South Africa's history and continues to cast a shadow over national politics. Mbeki argued that racism pervades mainstream scientific accounts of HIV in that they ascribe the severity of the epidemic in Africa to the supposedly deviant sexual conduct of black Africans. By drawing attention to the ways in which racism has supposedly corrupted Western HIV science, Mbeki and his supporters figured it as 'bad' science. In contrast, they depicted indigenous African knowledge about HIV/AIDS as 'good' science; that is, science capable of addressing the specificities of the HIV epidemic in Africa. While many scholars have dismissed the government's account of HIV as 'denialist' and therefore illegitimate, the material analysed here invites a somewhat different conclusion. It suggests that, although the government's approach was manifestly problematic and had far-reaching effects on South Africa's epidemic, it is also comprehensible within South Africa's specific circumstances and, indeed, it has historical resonance in light of South Africa's long history of racial oppression and colonialism. The echoes of this history reverberate in the gendered and racialised contours of the HIV epidemic in South Africa. For example, as we saw, the vestiges of institutionalised racism intra-act with racially uneven development, violent masculinities and unequal gender relations to produce the 'face' of the South African epidemic as predominantly female, black and poor.

Although Mbeki sidelined the issue of gender and its connection to HIV, he did make the legitimate observation that HIV in Africa is a disease of poverty. Yet this observation seems to have been swept aside by the intensified biomedical approach to addressing HIV. As Craddock puts it, 'the incontrovertible dominance of biomedical models placing HIV front and center have silenced Mbeki's more insightful comments on poverty's role in creating the South African epidemic' (2004, p. 5). In the presumed polarisation of the debate, the potentially helpful elements of Mbeki's dissident position were lost, incorporated under the rubric of 'denialism' and thus relegated to the terrain of non-science. However, a careful mapping of the accounts of science produced in the debate discloses considerable unacknowledged overlap in both parties' enactment of 'good' science. The substance of these overlapping views is, however, open to critique, both for its assumptions and for the role these assumptions played in constituting the epidemic. By charting the shared terrain in the TAC's and the government's accounts, my analysis has tried to avoid uncritically reproducing the presumed polarisation of the debate. Instead it has explored the generative work of the debate – and its depiction as starkly split – in constituting HIV in South Africa. If the presumed bifurcation of the debate had been more vigorously queried at the time, as the preceding discussion has attempted to do, and attention drawn to the shared ground in both parties' approaches to HIV, a rapprochement between the Mbeki government and the TAC could have developed and, with it, a more collaborative and thus effective approach to addressing HIV.

While important similarities in both parties' accounts of science can be observed, there are also points of difference in their accounts. For example, in contrast to the government's scepticism of the scientific orthodoxy on HIV, TAC's account of science seems to require a precritical adherence to Western science and its facts. This will not do either, practically or epistemologically. The Mbeki government's resistance to scientific orthodoxy is enough to remind us that conventional facts will not solve the HIV epidemic. HIV/AIDS cannot be accounted for by traditional scientific facts but it also exceeds the government's attempts to historicise and politicise these facts. Put in terms of the explanations offered in the debate, AIDS cannot be understood simply as a syndrome caused by a virus, nor merely as a symptom of structural factors such as poverty and racial differences, which appear resistant to change. Both explanations oversimplify this continually changing disease, reducing it to a fixed and stable object that the right kind of science can uncover. So how then might an agential realist refiguring of HIV change anything? Most obviously, it yields a different set of questions about prevention and treatment. Instead of asking, for example, *Why has condom usage (as the centrepiece of South Africa's prevention campaign) not been taken up uniformly?*, it might be more helpful to ask, *How can prevention strategies take account of patterns of concurrent sexual partnerships, and the history, gender norms and politics embodied in these patterns?* Or *How do diverse sexual practices and calculations of sexual risk intra-act with prevention strategies to compromise the latter's effectiveness?* The intensification of biomedical approaches to addressing HIV also prompts the question: *In their encounters with embodied subjects, what new material-discursive phenomena will biotechnologies such as ART help to generate?*

To return to Latour's insights, policy that treats HIV as a 'matter of concern' has the potential to disrupt the illusory biomedical/social, science/politics distinctions that have dominated conventional approaches to the problem, including the South African approach. Instead of prioritising behavioural over biomedical responses, or vice versa, policy animated by this alternative agenda treats the behavioural and biomedical as always already entangled and, crucially, it treats the facts of disease as made in part through policy itself. Attending to the multiple practices that jointly make HIV may enable the design of more effective, responsible policy. The term 'responsible' is intended to designate policy that is capable of recognising its contributory role in materialising HIV in specific and sometimes unintended ways. This would require some consideration of the material-discursive practices (including those associated with policy) that have produced damaging formations of the disease, such as those that connect HIV with sexual shame, negative stereotypes and discrimination. Such a policy agenda would also recognise that variations in policy responses to HIV produce qualitatively different disease epidemics in different demographic groups and geographical locations. Mapping these differently constituted epidemics in terms of the practices that produce them has the potential to enable policy-makers to engage the complexity of HIV's variation both within South Africa and across sub-Saharan Africa, as the region most affected by the HIV epidemic globally.

3
Poverty in the Making of HIV/AIDS

It is well-established that poverty and disease are intimately connected, with poverty often viewed as both a cause and consequence of disease. However, the nature and implications of this causal connection are understood in strikingly different ways in scientific and social studies of disease, each of which tend to posit disease as either biological or social in origin and thus accord varying degrees of primacy to the role of poverty – as a putatively social problem – in the aetiology and effects of disease. This chapter revisits the question of how poverty and disease are related, but does so in a way that avoids sequestering the biological dimensions of disease from its social dimensions. The starting point for my analysis is the Mbeki government's theory that AIDS is a disease of poverty and not simply the outcome of a viral infection. This account of AIDS supports a view of disease as the product of social forces. HIV activists in South Africa's Treatment Action Campaign (TAC) contested the government's claim that AIDS in Africa is a disease of poverty, arguing that poverty is a distal factor that shapes the disease but not its primary causal agent. Endorsing the orthodox scientific explanation, the TAC insisted that AIDS is caused by the virus HIV. In the framing of the TAC–government struggle, these two accounts of AIDS causation were treated as polarised along orthodox/dissident lines. But need they be viewed as mutually incompatible? Is it possible to treat AIDS as the outcome of a viral infection ('biology') *and* the product of poverty ('society')? And if so, what might be gained from doing so? Conversely, what is lost by holding fast to explanations that insist on a rigid distinction between the biological and social origins of disease? Against the commonplace view that the accounts of AIDS offered by the TAC and the Mbeki government were irreconcilably different, this chapter draws attention to an important (and concerning) similarity they share. Both accounts treat AIDS as a matter of fact: a fixed object that is either the product of biology (a viral infection) or the product of society (poverty). In what follows, I argue that disease exceeds any notion of simple fact, whether facts are construed as effects of biological or social forces.

The dynamics of AIDS and poverty: complicating conventional causal logic

> I came to the conclusion that as Africans we are confronted by a health crisis of enormous proportions. One of the consequences of this crisis is the deeply disturbing phenomenon of the collapse of immune systems among millions of our people, such that their bodies have no natural defence against attack by many viruses and bacteria [...] As I listened and heard the whole story told about our own country, it seemed to me that we could not blame everything on a single virus [HIV].
>
> It seemed to me also that every living African, whether in good or ill health, is prey to many enemies of health that would interact one upon the other in many ways, within one human body. (Mbeki, 2000d)

As is evident in his speech (quoted above) at the opening of the Thirteenth International HIV/AIDS conference, Mbeki did not dismiss HIV as among the causes of AIDS in Africa. However, he contested the prevailing scientific view that AIDS has a single, underlying viral cause and instead argued that AIDS is caused by a variety of interacting social, environmental and biological forces, figured via the metaphor of 'enemies of health' (Mbeki, 2000d). By depicting 'enemies of health' as forces that interact 'one upon the other' to produce illness, Mbeki's formulation posits the existence of discrete objects that impact independently on one another generating predictable effects on the individual 'human body'. These effects include a collapsed immune system (or in biomedical terms, AIDS), which prevents the body from defending itself against viruses or bacteria, and thus hinders its capacity to stave off illness. According to this view, disease is the predictable result of discrete but interacting causal factors ('enemies of health'), such as 'poor nutrition, unavailability of clean water, unhygienic environmental conditions, [the] unaffordability of drugs' and, 'inadequate [...] health services and infrastructure' (Mbeki, 2000a).

The TAC presents a somewhat similar account of the connection between poverty and HIV, proposing that poverty is both 'a cause and consequence of HIV-infection' (TAC Science and Research Committee, 2001, p. 38). In doing so, it acknowledges the two-way traffic between HIV and poverty:

Poverty contributing directly to the epidemic:

Particular groups are vulnerable to the disease as a consequence of their living without adequate means [...] Poverty also indirectly contributes to this epidemic and other diseases by causing poor physical health of people as well as through people's reduced control over circumstances. Limited access to education and information reduces the ability of many people in poverty to respond adequately to threats to their existence.

[...]

Poverty resulting from the epidemic:

Certain households face the prospect of poverty purely because they lose a breadwinner, need to care for sick family members, or have to take care of relatives from other households. There is therefore a specific need to address poverty that results from the disease itself. (TAC Science and Research Committee, 2001, pp. 38–39, original emphasis)

As noted above, TAC proposes a model of disease causation in which poverty is understood to be both a cause and effect of HIV: not only does poverty enhance vulnerability to HIV infection, it is also a consequence of HIV insofar as illness or death from HIV pushes households into poverty. Where the account articulated by Mbeki implies a unidirectional conception of poverty as a cause of HIV, TAC's account suggests the relationship between poverty and HIV is bidirectional. On this view, poverty is both a cause and effect of HIV. Yet despite this difference in their understanding of HIV causation, both TAC and the government treat poverty and HIV/AIDS as separate entities that interact with each other in linear ways to generate predictable effects. However, HIV and poverty can also be conceived in more relational terms as imbricated or enfolded in each other such that they defy explanation using simple 'cause and effect' logic. Exceeding both the unidirectional and bidirectional models of causation articulated above, we might productively understand the HIV–poverty dynamic as multidirectional, recursive and, perhaps most importantly, one in which HIV and poverty are ontologically entangled phenomena, rather than separately determinate entities. Reconceived this way, disease emerges as a multiply co-constituted phenomenon, formed through its encounters with other phenomena such as poor nutrition, inadequate health care and low levels of education (themselves co-constituted). I am suggesting, in other words, that disease embodies what is usually seen as its environment. According to this conceptualisation, when so-called environmental or social conditions change so too does the substance – the very materiality – of disease. As I go on to show, this alternative account has significant material implications for how the problem of HIV takes shape and, in turn, for the measures proposed to address it.

In order to make an argument about the co-constitution of disease and its environment, it is necessary to examine more closely the government and TAC's understandings of the relationship between HIV and poverty. I begin by analysing the government's argument that virological explanations for AIDS medicalise poverty, demonstrating its role in dividing disease into two apparently distinct domains – the biological and the social – which it assumes can be dealt with separately. My analysis draws attention to the significance of this division for the making of HIV/AIDS in South Africa.

HIV/AIDS and the 'medicalisation of poverty'

One of the key documents elucidating Mbeki's position on AIDS and poverty is a lengthy essay entitled 'Castro Hlongwane, Caravans, Cats, Geese, Foot and Mouth and Statistics: HIV/AIDS and the Struggle for the Humanisation of the African' (Anonymous, 2002). As noted in Chapter 2, this 114-page essay, which was circulated among the African National Congress (ANC) executive, is believed to have been written by ANC chief electoral officer Peter Mokaba, with assistance from Mbeki (Shisana and Simbayi, 2002). In Chapter 3, the authors lament what they see as the inadequacies of a medicalised approach to addressing 'Africa's health challenges':

> Stridently and openly, the omnipotent apparatus[1] disapproves of our effort seriously to deal with the serious challenge in our country of health, poverty and underdevelopment [...] According to this argument, necessarily, therefore, the two principal and decisive responses open to us, to respond to Africa's health challenges, are the use of condoms and the consumption of anti-retroviral drugs. Everything else that causes ill health and death among us, the omnipotent

apparatus argues, is of peripheral importance. (Anonymous, 2002, Chapter 3)

A couple of issues are collapsed in this passage that would benefit from being teased out. The authors critique the two central planks of the dominant biomedical response to HIV: (1) behavioural change measures, notably the promotion of condom use to prevent HIV transmission, and (2) anti-retroviral (ARV) drugs, which are currently the most effective form of HIV treatment. They argue that by prioritising the use of condoms and anti-retroviral drugs as the 'principal...responses...to Africa's health challenges', the international AIDS orthodoxy (or, to use the authors' rather more conspiratorial terms, 'the omnipotent apparatus') is annexing broader problems of poverty and underdevelopment in Africa under the biomedical umbrella of HIV/AIDS (Anonymous, 2002, Chapter 3).

Later, in Chapter 12 the authors revisit this theme:

one purpose they [Africans] serve for those who fatten them, is to medicalise poverty and underdevelopment. Thus problems that require a determined global effort to end African poverty and underdevelopment are presented, with African acquiescence, as problems that can be solved with condoms and drugs. (Anonymous, 2002, Chapter 12)

Both extracts contest the promotion of behavioural and biomedical strategies for managing HIV/AIDS on the basis that they medicalise the problem. The term 'medicalise' would benefit from a brief definition here. To medicalise something is to place it under the aegis of medicine and therefore understand it as responsive to medical intervention. The term first emerged in the 1970s in the social scientific literature and has generally been used to critique the increasing dominance of biomedical approaches in understanding and addressing disease, managing 'health risks' and optimising human life (Conrad, 1992; Persson, 2013). According to proponents of the medicalisation critique, the 'increasing power of scientific medicine [...] has detrimental effects for traditionally disempowered and exploited social groups by deflecting questions of social inequality into the realm of illness and disease, there to be treated inappropriately by drugs and other medical therapies' (Lupton, 1997, p. 96).

By claiming that the international AIDS establishment ('the omnipotent apparatus') medicalises diseases of poverty in Africa, the government resists what it sees as misguided attempts to place the problem of poverty within the province of medicine, to be solved through biomedical treatments. Essentially, the Mbeki government's medicalisation critique presents an argument against an exclusively biomedical response to HIV/AIDS on the basis that it does not address the disease's social causes and is driven only by sinister drug profiteering (an attempt to 'fatten Africans'). While recognising that this dualistic framing helped the government to advance their AIDS dissident position and their emphasis on addressing poverty and underdevelopment as key causes of disease, it also displaced from view more moderate understandings of disease causation that may have been expressed outside the polarised rhetoric of the debate. Importantly, by implicitly casting the social as distinct from and counter to the biomedical, the medicalisation critique retains the traditional dualism (and its implicit hierarchy) of biomedical/social knowledge. The government's reliance on this dualism, and its associated attempt to quarantine the social domains of HIV from medical ones is not merely an epistemological issue; it generated some real and damaging effects. For one, by treating the cause of HIV as reducible to poverty and rejecting the accepted medical explanation, the government sidelined existing biomedical technologies to treat those already infected and focused instead on social and behavioural responses. Partly because of its concerns about the toxicity of ARV drugs, South Africa's government under Mbeki refused to deliver anti-retroviral therapy (ART) as part of its national HIV treatment strategy. Only in late 2003, when a court order compelled it to do so, did the Health Ministry implement a national ART programme.

The separation of social and medical knowledge about disease is common, but as the South African case reveals, it is not only conceptually shaky but also materially harmful. In the case of HIV, the stakes are very high: during the period of Mbeki's presidency, an estimated 300,000 people, reliant on public health care, died from treatable AIDS-related illnesses (Chigwedere *et al.*, 2008). In Barad's agential realist terms, we can understand these deaths as produced through the intra-actions of HIV, the state of South Africa's public health care system, the reliance upon a medical/social dualism in understanding the disease's causes, AIDS dissidence, an inadequate national HIV policy, antagonistic relations between the state and local AIDS activist organisations including the TAC, reduced public health spending on HIV and other so-called political forces usually seen as separate from, if not irrelevant to, AIDS-related mortality. Moreover, the government's reliance on a biomedical/social dualism arguably deflected attention away from other important intra-actions shaping HIV/AIDS in South Africa, such as regional politicking and Mbeki's neoliberal economic policy, which was inconsistent with his professed concern to alleviate poverty (Decoteau, 2013).

In making this argument I am not of course suggesting, following a conventional causal logic, that any of these phenomena can be singled out as a separately determinate 'cause' of the deaths from AIDS (the 'effect'). Rather, my point is that these phenomena and the deaths emerge in relation to each other. They make (and, sometimes, change) each other in their encounters and are therefore ontologically entangled. The deaths from AIDS, for example, arguably helped to entrench the antagonistic relations between the state and local AIDS activist organisations, thus impeding action on HIV treatment and enabling more AIDS-related deaths. The deaths are also likely to have confirmed the inadequacies of the public health system and Mbeki's HIV policy, deepening the public's lack of confidence in the already struggling public health sector (Harris et al., 2011) and quite possibly discouraging HIV-positive people from seeking care. In short, the high AIDS mortality rate under Mbeki is both materially shaped by and shapes these key political phenomena.

By pointing out some of the limitations of the government's focus on so-called social strategies to combat HIV/AIDS (poverty alleviation and behavioural change measures), I am not suggesting that an exclusively biomedical response is the answer either. In order to gauge the effects of a predominantly medical response, it is helpful to examine TAC's approach to addressing HIV in South Africa.

Entangled ontologies: poverty in the making of HIV/AIDS

Responding to the government's argument that AIDS is a disease of poverty, TAC leaders supported the biomedical model of AIDS causation, arguing that 'Only HIV predicts AIDS [...] No other factor on its own, including drug use, diet or poverty, is sufficient to cause AIDS' (Geffen, 2006, p. 2). As this statement illustrates, it instated a hierarchy in which poverty was treated as a distal factor contributing to AIDS, but not its primary causal agent. By privileging the virological explanation for AIDS, the TAC reinforced the long-standing biologically determinist view that biology (in this case, a viral infection) precedes and is the foundation for other social causes of disease (for example, 'drug use, diet or poverty'). Coupling a biomedical account with a pro-poor treatment movement, the organisation focused on one aspect of poverty as crucial to combating HIV/AIDS, namely access to health care.

TAC leader Nathan Geffen explains the connection between poverty and AIDS in the following terms, pointing out what he sees as an important oversight in Mbeki's formulation:

> There is one particularly crucial way in which poverty exacerbates Aids [sic] that Mbeki almost entirely ignored [...] Poor people do not have access to the health services of the well-off [...] Until ARVs and other medicines for opportunistic infections were widely available in the public health system – and even since – the poor died of Aids [sic] in large numbers in South Africa precisely because it was much more difficult for them than for well-off people with medical insurance to get ARVs. (Geffen, 2010, pp. 28–9)

This statement frames the connection between poverty and AIDS narrowly, focusing on access to affordable medical treatment and sidelining the role of other poverty-related phenomena in shaping vulnerability to HIV/AIDS, such as unemployment, food insecurity, limited access to sanitation facilities, makeshift housing conditions and malnutrition. In so doing, it elevates the importance of biomedical measures (drugs) in addressing HIV and reduces the significance of other measures. Of course, such a response is understandable given the insufficiency of the government's approach, particularly its refusal to deliver ART. It is also worth noting that, once HIV treatment became available in South Africa's public health system, TAC shifted their focus from treatment access to treatment literacy programmes, which address the role of nutrition, access to safe drinking water and other poverty-related factors in managing HIV/AIDS (Peacock *et al.*, 2008). This suggests that TAC is cognizant of the multiple factors that shape the relations of poverty and HIV in South Africa, but this more nuanced understanding of the poverty–HIV dynamic drops out of view in the above account, which emphasises instead the absence of medical treatment in aggravating poverty and AIDS. With this in mind, it seems that the explanatory narrowness of the conception articulated here was at least in part an effect of the polarised HIV debate and the manifest inadequacies of the Mbeki government's HIV policy approach. In short, my concern here is not simply to point out the limitations of either the government's or TAC's approach (as others have done). Rather, it is to show how the politics of the debate – and its presumed polarisation – impacted materially on the measures taken to address HIV in South Africa, and therefore on the epidemic itself.

Intriguing, though, is Geffen's qualification that, *even since* ARVs have been publicly available, the poor have continued to die from AIDS. If access to drugs, in particular ARVs, is the definitive factor governing the continued association of AIDS with poverty in South Africa, then why has access not resulted in a decoupling of poverty and AIDS-related mortality? Perhaps the answer can be found in a rethinking of the relations of poverty, AIDS and ARV drugs. Geffen's statement presumes that poverty, AIDS and ARV drugs are separate, autonomous entities that impact on each other in predictable ways. But they can also be understood as co-constitutive phenomena, made and transformed in their relations. This different conception of the poverty–disease–drugs dynamic entails a rethinking of intervention. Instead of thinking of poverty and HIV/AIDS as subject *to* intervention and ARVs as the tool *of* intervention, we might usefully conceive poverty and HIV as already an effect of intervention (Rosengarten, 2009). Such a reconception invites consideration of the role of interventions themselves (as part of a larger relational field) in making and changing the disease. The pursuit of such reflexive measures has the potential to prevent those working in the field of HIV from proceeding as though they are merely *responding* to the disease – as if it were a transparently given object that precedes attempts to treat it using biotechnologies such as ARVs. It opens up possibilities for *intra-acting* with HIV as an emergent, agentive phenomenon that is changed by, and helps to change, particular treatment measures and technologies themselves.

In arguing for the generative role of interventions, I am not discounting the work of ARVs in treating HIV but rather arguing that ARVs do not intervene in a direct, linear way on their 'target'. Instead, they help to constitute the virus, just as ARVs themselves are constituted in their encounters with the virus. For example, and as noted in the previous chapter, the fact that HIV can mutate into drug-resistant strains when a person takes ART irregularly or stops treatment highlights the role of ARV drugs in materially shaping the virus. Here variability in HIV is contingent on specific treatment technologies, viral replication and irregular dosing or cessation of ARV drugs. ARV drugs are also changed in these encounters, rendered less effective or even ineffective in treating emerging drug-resistant strains of the virus. As this example makes clear, HIV and specific treatment technologies are made and changed in their encounters, challenging the assumption that the virus exists independently of and anterior to the measures designed to treat it. In other words, and following Rosengarten and Michael (2009), we can say that

HIV and ARV drugs actively (and multiply) produce each other and therefore cannot be considered singular, bounded entities that merely interact in predictable ways.

Of central interest here is the role of multiple phenomena in shaping the ways in which HIV/AIDS and poverty are connected. So the continued deaths of poor people from AIDS, even in the presence of treatment, should prompt consideration of the larger relational field that helps to (re)produce poverty's association with the disease. To explore what this field might look like, I examine Geffen's explanation of the link between AIDS and poverty, where he cites the example of an HIV-positive man living in a township in Cape Town:

> [HIV-positive] Andile Madondile took me to his tiny shack in Khayelitsha [a township in Cape Town], which he shares with his wife and two children.[2] There is barely any privacy [...] There is no tap in Andile's shack. The one a few metres from it was vandalised by *tsotsis* [young urban criminals] and Andile's ward councillor has not done anything to repair it despite promising to do so. So the nearest tap is about 100 metres from his shack. The nearest toilet is even further. His shack, the tap and toilet make a triangle of inconvenient town-planning with devastating public health consequences. How is poverty related to Aids? [sic] For one thing, as Andile's circumstances show, it makes day-to-day living with the virus and opportunistic infections difficult. Diarrhoea is a part of life in the advanced stages of HIV. (Geffen, 2010, p. 27)

According to Geffen, Andile's situation demonstrates a causal chain between circumstances of poverty and AIDS-related illness: the location of sanitation and clean drinking water far from Andile's shack cause 'devastating public health consequences', including AIDS-related illnesses, such as diarrhoea. Poverty is also seen as exacerbating the effects of these illnesses by 'making day-to-day living with [...] opportunistic infections difficult' (Geffen, 2010, p. 27). On this reading, it is possible to infer that, all other things being equal, if Andile were living in more affluent conditions, he might not experience AIDS-related illness or at least it would not be as debilitating. It is interesting that, of the factors that could be said to cause Andile's illness, Geffen singles out the location of his shack in relation to the tap and toilet, describing it as a 'triangle of inconvenient town-planning'. However, Andile's illness can also be seen as emerging in relation to a complex assemblage of phenomena that includes, but is not limited to, the location of his shack. Some of these phenomena are mentioned in the extract above and some can be inferred from the fuller account of Andile's story told earlier in Geffen's book. They include HIV, unemployment, malnutrition, the decision not to take ARVs, dense informal housing, the effects of vandalism in the township, poor municipal management and the location of flush toilets and clean water. In their intra-actions, these phenomena constitute Andile's AIDS-related illness and are themselves reconstituted. The dynamic process of intra-activity outlined in this example complicates assumptions about a neat causal relationship between the apparently discrete entities of AIDS and poverty. Furthermore, the notion of intra-activity illuminates Andile's illness as embodying (rather than simply caused by) poverty-related phenomena. So the diarrhoea Andile experiences can be understood not simply as the product of an AIDS-related opportunistic infection (although the infection and Andile's HIV status are important factors) but as a product of the phenomenon of poverty. It is, therefore, possible to see AIDS as a qualitatively different disease when it is materialised in poor, under-resourced settings than when it is materialised in comparatively affluent, well-resourced ones. This is not to suggest that, as in the conventional reading, poverty merely contributes to hastening the onset of AIDS, or that it exacerbates its symptoms, but rather that it is integral to the ontology of the disease in South Africa. In other words, the disease cannot be separated from its relational context; it is formed and re-formed through it.

On the basis of this re-reading of the dynamics of AIDS and poverty, it should come as no surprise that, despite the availability of ARVs in the South African public sector, the symbolic-material association between the disease and poverty persists. One of the effects of this enduring association is that, as Geffen notes, many poor South Africans continue to die from AIDS. Treating HIV/AIDS with ARV drugs will not by itself solve the problem of HIV in South Africa as it fails to address the co-constituted problem of poverty. My intention here is not to dismiss the significance of ART in addressing the epidemic but rather to question the emphasis that has been placed on it and the associated tendency to de-accent approaches that tackle the social-behavioural dimensions of disease. Resonating with this concern about the effects of an intensified biomedical treatment approach, medical anthropologists Margaret Lock and Vinh-Kim Nguyen (2010, p. 156) note that '[j]uggernaut AIDS treatment programs, with their focus on saving individual lives through treatment, have effectively moved the response away from an emphasis on social determinants and even away from prevention programs to focus on biology alone'.

It may sound paradoxical but a narrow clinical orientation to HIV (and the associated bracketing out of social, political and economic issues) can have a detrimental impact on the delivery of clinical treatment measures themselves. For example, HIV treatment can be rendered less effective by poverty-related phenomena such as food insecurity, poor sanitation and limited access to health care (Leclerc-Madlala, 2006). Treatment uptake and compliance are also detrimentally affected by under-resourced, rural conditions where people have limited mobility to regularly access and therefore adhere to treatment, as is the case in many South African settings (Robins, 2009). Another apparently external factor impacting on the effectiveness of ART in South Africa is the ongoing shortage of two types of ARV medicines (tenofovir and abacavir) in clinics across the country (TAC, 2012). These shortages can interrupt ART, creating the conditions for drug-resistant strains of HIV to develop. Currently, no policy is in place to prevent drug shortages or to advise clinics on the different combinations of drugs that can be administered if one type of ARV is unavailable (Bateman, 2013; TAC, 2012). And even in cases where clinics are equipped to provide a different combination of ART, prolonged use of the alternative medication (stavudine) is associated with debilitating side-effects, 'increased rates of non-adherence and consequent treatment failure' (South African Clinicians Society, 2012, p. 1). I argue that these forces shape the virus and HIV treatment in real and significant ways. Perhaps most obviously, drug shortages, in their encounters with HIV patients, individual viral load counts, drug side-effects and treatment interruptions, help to transform the virus. In the process, ARVs too are transformed, rendered less effective or even ineffective in combating the new drug-resistant forms of the virus. As more drug-resistant forms of HIV emerge, the range of available treatment combinations is reduced, making HIV more difficult to treat, and requiring new drugs.

In drawing attention to key phenomena that can help render ART less effective or ineffective, it might appear that, like Mbeki, I am making an argument against ART, one that could reduce political commitment to a national ART programme in South Africa. This, of course, is not my aim. Rather, I am seeking to demonstrate that socio-political phenomena such as poverty, drug shortages and poorly managed ART provision are integral to the constitution of HIV. The disease does not precede political and social practices; it is made and remade within them. As we have seen, when HIV is made (or changed), so too is its treatment. Therefore, when socio-political phenomena are positioned low in the hierarchy of HIV treatment (and indeed considered distinct from medical concerns), the success of treatment itself is seriously undermined. Social, political and cultural forces are not usually recognised as being central to a scientific conception of disease but, as I have demonstrated, disease always already embodies socio-political concerns. To treat these as separate from the medico-scientific enterprise is to impoverish science and diminish our capacity to address destructive disease epidemics, such as the HIV epidemic. In short, I argue that effective responses to HIV will be better served by understanding the ontology of disease as emergent, produced in the intra-actions of social, political and biological forces.

Victims and vectors of disease

As discussed in Chapter 2, ideas about disease help to constitute not only the disease itself but also those affected by it (often described as the 'targets' of disease). In other words, disease and its 'targets' emerge in relation to each other or, in agential realist terms, they materialise in their intra-actions. In what follows I trace some of these intra-actions, showing how HIV and affected individuals are forged not only in their relations with each other, but also in their encounters with treatment, poverty, ideas about HIV transmission, and the normative ideals of public health. In doing so, I address one of the key questions underpinning this book: what kinds of subjects do particular materialisations of HIV help to produce?

By presenting poverty as a necessary partner to HIV/AIDS, the Mbeki government implied that the poor are more vulnerable to HIV infection. Consequently, poor people were the target of the government's HIV prevention strategies and this arguably served to doubly stigmatise them as victims of poverty *and* disease. This framing may reinforce associations already drawn between poor people, inadequate living conditions and malnutrition, instating a view of the poor as disease carriers. Yet, as the case of a country like Australia demonstrates, the association of HIV with poverty is entirely circumstantial. Australia has a concentrated HIV epidemic, almost entirely restricted to men who have sex with men and poverty is not identified as a determining factor in new infections (Guy *et al.*, 2007). As this comparison shows, the assumed causal relationship between HIV and poverty in South Africa is not inevitable. It is contingent on specific historical, social and political arrangements that are amenable to change, which means that the association between HIV and poverty can be undone (or at least loosened), challenging the negative stereotype that poor people are disease vectors. This shift in thinking about HIV may open up a broader range of responses that address the prevalence of the disease across the socioeconomic spectrum, rather than as the inevitable product of poverty. A change in responses transforms the disease itself and, in some cases, the epidemiology of the epidemic.

Although I have argued that poverty helps to produce specific ontologies of HIV in South Africa, treating the disease as largely a symptom of poverty overlooks the fact that people across the socioeconomic spectrum can become infected with HIV. Therefore, public health messages that uncritically reproduce the association of HIV with poverty could create the conditions for new infections to spread among more affluent populations, who may perceive their risk of contracting the virus to be low (Tladi, 2006). This is at least partly because judgements of HIV risk are made not simply on the basis of biomedical knowledge about HIV, but also according to normative judgements about a prospective sexual partner's risk profile, including characteristics associated with 'high-risk' stereotypes and known or assumed HIV status (Race, 2001). On this reading, it is possible to understand individual risk calculus as embodying estimates of epidemiological risk and public health messages that equate HIV with poverty. Instead of understanding these informational aspects (risk estimates and public health messages) as pre-existing, separate 'tools' for intervening to prevent HIV infection, it is worth considering what might be gained by treating them as dynamic phenomena that *intra-act* with the 'targets of prevention' to produce an altered and potentially harmful sexual risk calculus. Where the conventional view of public health strategies aimed at lowering HIV risk instates a distinction between information and matter and 'installs a given and therefore normative conception of human agency as distinct from the matter that it is affecting and affected by', the refigured conception proposed here posits information and matter as co-constituted (Rosengarten, 2009, p. 61). Such a refiguring is important for at least three reasons:

1. It allows for a more nuanced understanding of, and thus a more effective engagement with the dynamic relational field of HIV in which 'socio-sexual subjects' participate and take calculated sexual risks (Race, 2001, p. 171).
2. It enables a richer account of the 'targets' of prevention as constitutive of their environment and as helping to change this environment. Agency, on this post-humanist view, is not confined to human subjects; it is distributed across the relational field of HIV. According

Poverty in the Making of HIV/AIDS 81

to a distributed notion of agency, prevention measures directed at responsible/irresponsible human subjects fail to address the complex matrix of human and non-human practices through which HIV is produced, and in which prevention practices themselves participate (Rosengarten, 2009).

3. Related to the point above, recognising the coextensive relation between disease concepts and the materiality of disease allows for consideration of the role of policy and public health messages in shaping the very substance of HIV. It opens up the possibility of advancing more effective treatment and prevention measures, responsive to the ways in which the measures themselves participate in making (and changing) HIV.

To return to the government's understanding of the relationship between HIV and poverty, it is worth noting, at this point, that Mbeki's construction of HIV/AIDS as a disease of poverty was arguably an attempt to break another harmful symbolic-material association: that between HIV and sexual promiscuity. In August 2000, South African journalist Mark Gevisser raised the issue of AIDS-related stigma in an interview with Mbeki, asking why he thought that many public figures living with HIV did not disclose their HIV status. Mbeki's response is framed within a discourse of sexual shame, reinforcing prejudices that link HIV to sexual promiscuity:

> If I stood up tomorrow and said, 'I am HIV-positive', the assumption would be that the president has been sleeping with prostitutes! And I suppose that no one would want to be identified like that! (Mbeki, 2000, cited in Gevisser, 2009, p. 294)

According to Gevisser, Mbeki then went on to explain that identifying poverty as a cause of HIV does not invoke the same stigma. Mbeki implies that endorsing this alternative causal explanation would help to destigmatise HIV, thus potentially facilitating greater acceptance of those affected. Importantly, the distinction Mbeki makes between the causal agents of HIV (sexual transmission versus poverty) is about where responsibility for the disease is presumed to lie. According to Mbeki, the public tends to view individuals who contract HIV through so-called risky sexual practices ('sleeping with prostitutes') as blameworthy, and by implication they presume that prostitutes are disease vectors. By contrast, those who contract HIV as a result of poverty, malnutrition and limited access to health care are likely to be seen as innocent victims of structural conditions that make them more susceptible to disease.

The distinction drawn here between vehicles of HIV transmission identifies a moral hierarchy of innocence/guilt located in the HIV-positive subject. Not only do these attributions make normative moral judgements, they also assume a hard-and-fast distinction between individual and structural factors that contribute to disease: whereas sexual practices are assumed to be within an individual's control, structural factors such as poverty are deemed outside their control. Assumptions about individual versus structural culpability produce different understandings of the causation of HIV. As already noted, where the causal link between HIV and poverty is emphasised and that between HIV and particular sexual practices is de-emphasised, it could contribute to the dangerous misconception that only poor people are vulnerable to infection. Furthermore, the assumption that poverty is a structural problem, outside individual control, implies that the concurrence of HIV and poverty is inevitable: hence HIV infection is unavoidable among this demographic. Although one obviously cannot neglect the role of poverty in shaping HIV and its subjects, it is possible that such a view could contribute to new infections by generating a sense of fatalism among those living in poverty and those who advocate for them. In other words, and in contrast to the biomedical model and its emphasis on individual agency and volition, Mbeki's approach decentres volitional action by foregrounding the role of poverty in shaping vulnerability to HIV. Furthermore, given that prostitution is often closely associated with poverty, it makes little sense to separate the two. Instead, these putative disease 'vectors' are subject to the same forces as impoverished 'victims'.

The point here is that ideas like Mbeki's about the causation of HIV do not *reflect* a pre-existing reality of the disease; through their iteration, these ideas partake in *constituting* the disease and those affected by it. This is a crucial distinction because much is at stake in how HIV is variously made and transformed. Where HIV is produced as inevitably arising from circumstances of poverty, the strategies chosen to address it can reify and cement this causal link because they treat the association between HIV and poverty as natural or inevitable, rather than as contingent on particular ideas about disease. The government's emphasis on pursuing poverty alleviation strategies to combat HIV can therefore be seen as reproducing, rather than disrupting, the symbolic-material link between the disease and poverty in South Africa. Of course, other practices, relations and ideas about HIV also contribute to the material reproduction of this link. For example, as discussed, treating HIV/AIDS as poverty's inevitable consort may act as a disincentive to safe sex practices, enabling rates of infection to increase among the poor. We can therefore describe the concurrence of HIV and poverty in South Africa as partly an effect of particular disease concepts and policy approaches, rather than as natural or inevitable.

Furthermore, and as already noted, the causal link that Mbeki makes between HIV and poverty may help to reinforce a negative stereotype of poor people as disease vectors. Presenting HIV in these terms thus runs a similarly high risk of stigmatising a particular group as does the conventional view that it is a sexually transmitted disease. In this sense, Mbeki's formulation simply shifts the targets of stigma rather than removing the stigma entirely. It also shifts responsibility for HIV to those who are less able to advocate for themselves in the public sphere, unlike the wealthy and well-connected. Importantly, a view that posits HIV as the predictable result of poverty de-emphasises the role of sexual practices in the prevention and transmission of HIV. I am, of course, not suggesting that HIV infection is simply the outcome of 'risky' practices and all that is needed to combat infection is to stop people engaging in these practices. If it were this simple, behavioural change programmes would have been resoundingly successful in halting the spread of HIV. Nonetheless, in the network of relations within which HIV is formed (and transformed), sexual practices often play a significant role. De-accenting them – as Mbeki did – helped to impoverish the government's understanding of HIV, and diminish the effectiveness of its prevention strategies.

From helpless victims of HIV to agentive biological citizens

The TAC challenged the moralising basis of Mbeki's depiction of the HIV-positive subject, but in so doing, enacted their own versions which, as we will see, also produced some damaging effects. The TAC emphasised lack of access to affordable ART as being the main barrier to combating the epidemic and, more specifically, to mitigating its concentration among the poor. In a 2001 court case in which the government and TAC jointly challenged the Pharmaceutical Manufacturers' Association on the issue of patent abuse, TAC's lawyers framed the argument for affordable HIV treatment in life and death terms:

> It is not disputed that anti-retroviral drugs have now been developed which target HIV directly and significantly reduce the replication of

the virus, thereby preventing illness and the onset of AIDS [...] However, the cost of these anti-retroviral drugs in South Africa (between R2000 and R4000 per person per month) remains beyond the means of most persons living with HIV/AIDS.[3]

Thus, most South Africans living with HIV/AIDS are condemned to follow a path towards inevitable death over an average period of ten years from their infection. (Marcus and Shaskalson, 2001, paras 2.4 and 2.5)

This statement expresses the view that, in the absence of treatment, HIV-positive people can do nothing to maintain their health and stave off death. In the words of TAC's lawyers, affected individuals who cannot afford costly treatment in the private sector are 'condemned to follow a path towards inevitable death' (Marcus and Shaskalson, 2001, para. 2.5). Here, the HIV-positive subject is constituted as a helpless victim in three senses: a victim of a treatable disease, a victim of poverty and, perhaps most importantly, a victim of drug profiteering, which prevents access to life-prolonging treatment. Constructing HIV-positive individuals in these terms serves the legal strategy of emphasising the pressing need for affordable HIV treatment but it also strips them of agency. It is worth pointing out that this depiction of HIV-positive people is context specific: in TAC's health promotion literature (published once ART was available in the public health care system), those with HIV are consistently figured as agentive health consumers, rather than as victims of disease. Yet, given TAC's earlier depiction of people living with HIV as helpless victims, it seems questionable whether access to treatment alone can enable their transformation into powerful health consumers.

The figure of the HIV-positive subject as victim is also evident in the second court case in which the TAC was involved, where it challenged the government's approach to the prevention of mother-to-child transmission (PMTCT). At the time, South Africa's Health Ministry was piloting a phased approach to PMTCT. This approach meant that only a limited number of pregnant women attending clinics in the pilot sites would have access to PMTCT for the two-year duration of the pilot study, putting the unborn babies of women outside these sites at risk of infection. In 2001, after repeated unsuccessful attempts to persuade the government to deliver a national PMTCT programme, the TAC filed a lawsuit against the Minister of Health and the Provincial Health Departments arguing that their PMTCT policy was unconstitutional (Heywood, 2003). In presenting its heads of argument, TAC's legal counsel described the plight of babies born to HIV-positive women in the following terms:

> The devastating impact of HIV is borne out by the accounts of women who have been unable to obtain treatment to reduce the risk of transmission to their children and now have to live with the knowledge of the impending deaths of their offspring [...] Busisiwe Maqungo tested positive for HIV in May 1999 [...] At the time of her pregnancy she was aware that the drug AZT would reduce the risk of mother-to-child transmission of HIV. Notwithstanding the existence of this drug she gave birth to an HIV positive child without the advantage of this medication. In consequence, her baby is always sick and she has been told that her baby will die and that nothing can be done. (Marcus and Majola, 2001, paras 4.1–4.16)

This extract depicts women living with HIV as powerless to prevent their babies from contracting HIV, despite the existence of drugs that can reduce the risk of transmission. To underscore their powerlessness and the arbitrariness of the government's PMTCT policy, TAC's counsel goes on to argue that that these women who 'by reasons of poverty or geographical location are unable to receive the drug are simply left with no choice at all [...] their babies will be infected with HIV and will die a premature death' (Marcus and Majola, 2001, paras 5.13.12 and 15.14). As TAC member Busisiwe puts it, in terms that invite compassion for her plight: 'I gave birth to an HIV positive baby who should have been saved. That was my experience, the sad one, and I will live with it until my last day' (Maqungo, 2001, para. 16).

The image of the powerless victim relies for its force on the prevailing image of women and children as vulnerable and at increased risk of HIV infection. Moreover, because those at risk of HIV are unborn babies, they are construed as especially defenceless victims of a poorly formulated government policy. In this sense, we might describe the court case as enacting a hierarchy of victimhood where babies, by virtue of their vulnerability, are seen as in need of special protection. This enactment appeals to what sociologist Nicole Vitellone (2011, p. 580) has called an 'affective politics of compassion'. In this context, appeals to a politics of compassion serve to evoke sympathy for the helpless child. This affective politics also produces a hierarchy of innocence related to modes of HIV contraction. According to this hierarchy, babies who acquire HIV perinatally are considered to be 'entirely innocent' victims (Botha, 2001, p. 2). The binary logic of innocence/guilt implies that people who acquired HIV through other ways – for example through unprotected sex – bear more culpability for the acquisition and/or spread of the virus. Thus, it instates a moral politics centred on the dualisms of justice/injustice and innocence/guilt. This logic of innocence/guilt is part of the attraction of the poverty explanation which Mbeki endorsed: arguing that HIV is a disease of poverty suspends blame for HIV, whereas the orthodox explanation's emphasis on sexual practices attracts blame in that it presumes those who have HIV are culpable for acquiring and/or spreading the virus.

The moral politics of innocence/guilt invoked by the TAC helps to constitute a PMTCT programme as 'morally necessary' and constitutionally just on the grounds that it protects the lives of innocents (Kapczynski and Berger, 2009, p. 4). Indeed, when the legal judgment was delivered this moral politics was reinforced via reference to the 'entirely innocent' figure of the unborn child:

> The background to the application is the grim reality that 24% of pregnant women in South Africa are HIV positive and that 70 000 children are infected each year through MTCT [mother to child transmission] of HIV. It is one the most common forms of infection. It stands to reason that the *victim* of such a transmission is *entirely innocent*. (Botha, 2001, p. 2, emphasis added)

The privileged status accorded to babies who acquire HIV perinatally is illustrated by Busisiwe's poignant account of her initial decision to refuse treatment on the basis that her child had died without it: 'At first I didn't want treatment because my child who was innocent suffered and died without treatment and here I am healthy. She should not have suffered' (Maqungo, 2001, para. 13). Busisiwe's statement points to the material, political and ethical implications of defining HIV-positive individuals according to a binary logic of innocence/guilt: where a symbolic association is made between innocence/guilt and deserving/undeserving subjects, it operates to delineate HIV-positive individuals into two collectivities, those who are considered deserving of treatment and those who are considered less deserving (or even undeserving).

It is worth pointing out that this delineation is not merely hypothetical. During a parliamentary debate, a member of the opposition Inkatha Freedom Party made the distinction between more and less deserving subjects to argue for the rationing of HIV treatment to pregnant women, rape victims and health workers:

Treatment of mothers, to reduce by 50% the spread of HIV to infants, is an important issue. It is an issue of cost, practicality and ethics. If we cannot treat everyone, then whom do we treat? Surely pregnant women, rape victims and health workers are the most deserving. (Parliament of the Republic of South Africa, 2000, p. 35)

What do babies born to HIV-positive women, rape victims and health workers have in common that make them 'most deserving [of treatment]'? One likely answer is that they are perceived as having acquired HIV innocently: through an act of gender-based violence (rape victims), or a work-related injury (health workers) or perinatally (babies). Here distinctions between modes of HIV transmission that instate a binary logic of innocence/guilt, operate to constitute the babies of HIV-positive women, health workers and rape survivors as innocent victims of the disease and worthy recipients of treatment. At the same time, those who contracted/transmitted HIV through other means – for example, unprotected sex or sharing needles – are implicitly figured as guilty and less deserving of treatment. According to this reductive logic, individuals are *either* agentive in contracting or transmitting HIV (and are therefore culpable of harming themselves or others) *or* they are passive victims of forces beyond their control (in which case they are innocent). This binary framing obscures the multiple factors that contribute to the acquisition and spread of HIV, such as gendered inequalities that shape safe sex negotiations, the use of sex in exchange for money or food, widespread reliance on male condoms as a prevention technology, the limited political support for vaginal and anal microbicides as alternative prevention technologies and the availability of sterile injecting equipment (in the case of injecting drug use). The point here is that normalising assumptions regarding the culpability or innocence of particular groups in HIV acquisition and/or transmission can shape their access to treatment. In turn, the question of treatment access has a very important bearing on whether affected individuals live with HIV or die prematurely from AIDS.

As already mentioned, the TAC did not consistently construct HIV-positive subjects as victims of the government's poor policy decisions or as casualties of multinational pharmaceutical greed. The delivery of ART in the public health sector prompted a marked shift in the way in which people living with HIV were constituted via TAC's activist movement. Once ART was available, members of TAC redirected their advocacy efforts away from treatment access towards ensuring the successful delivery of ART and promoting treatment literacy (Peacock *et al.*,

2007). TAC's treatment literacy and health promotion literature published after the introduction of ART reveals a tendency to address people living with HIV as self-surveying biological citizens. The concept of 'biological citizenship' requires a brief definition here. First elaborated by prominent social theorist Nikolas Rose (2007), the term 'biological citizenship' is intended to capture the processes by which political projects have come to be articulated in biological terms. Part of the 'biologization of politics' or biopolitics, this new form of citizenship has meant that life itself has opened up as medium for the exercise of power and governmentality (Rose, 2007; Rose and Novas, 2005). In other words, as a mode through which biopolitics operates, biological citizenship entails a new understanding of how power and the body are related, one that addresses the productive disciplinary power of contemporary norms of health and the framing of citizens' rights and responsibilities in biological terms. In Western liberal democracies, the imperatives of biological citizenship can be seen in the emphasis on continual self-management, health optimisation and disease prevention. TAC's model of health citizenship is consistent with the biopolitics of contemporary Western liberal democracies because it too gives emphasis to self-management, health optimisation and disease prevention (Decoteau, 2013).

As with the depiction of the HIV-positive subject as a victim, it is my contention that the TAC did not merely *represent* those with HIV as biological citizens, it *constituted* them as such with rather mixed and uneven effects. To trace some of the effects, let us consider how HIV-positive subjects are constituted at the time of diagnosis in a TAC information booklet on living with HIV:

The first day

Perhaps you have just found out that you are HIV positive, and you are feeling shocked and scared. Learning that you are HIV positive can change your life, but there is a lot of help for you in South Africa. Here are a few steps that may help you plan and structure your life, now that you have been diagnosed.

Step 1

Take control! Go on with your life as best you can. Stay as busy as possible. Make a plan to get the best care and treatment possible. Learning all you can about HIV and the best treatment will give you more confidence. (Clayden *et al.*, 2013, p. 10)

Several elements are worth noting in this extract. First, the emphasis on planning and structuring one's life after receiving a diagnosis of HIV implants the imperative to enforce some kind of order on what would presumably be an otherwise unstructured or even chaotic response to an HIV-positive result. This advice embodies the logic of order/disorder, where order (or 'structure' in TAC's terms) is idealised and its presumed opposite, disorder, is seen as self-evidently problematic and therefore something to be overcome by following the consecutive steps set out in TAC's booklet. Given the onerous drug regimens associated with ART, the attempt to instate 'structure' in the life of a newly diagnosed HIV-positive person could be seen as prefiguring the requirement that they organise their life spatially and temporally around ART (Race, 2001).

Second, the strenuous expectation that the subject behave *proactively* ('Take control!) and *rationally* ('make a plan to get the best care and treatment possible') on receiving their HIV test results is arguably at odds with the acknowledgement that 'learning you are HIV-positive can change your life' (Clayden *et al*., 2013, p. 10). Indeed, it is possible to see the opposite kinds of behaviour – 'irrational' and 'passive/reactive' behaviour – as legitimate responses to receiving a potentially very distressing diagnosis that 'can change' one's life. Implicit here is the assumption that irrational or passive behaviour is not only undesirable, but also unstructured or disordered. Such behaviour needs correcting to conform to the structured response prescribed by the TAC. The imperative behind TAC's advice is not to accommodate what it construes as unstructured, and therefore undesirable behaviour, but to displace such behaviour altogether.

How is order/structure conceptualised here? Order (or, in TAC's terms, 'plan[ning] and structur[ing] your life') is understood to mean rational and agentive behaviour. As Fraser and Moore (2008) point out in an analysis of the order/disorder binary as it is enacted in a rather different context – that of injecting drug use – this conception of order is part of and helps to sustain a larger social order, the modern Western neoliberal order. Yet so-called unstructured or disordered conduct might usefully be refigured, not as the absence of order, but rather as the absence of a 'desired normative order' (Angelides, 2011, p. 16). This rethinking challenges the presumed undesirability of irrational and passive conduct. Crucially, it allows for the possibility that some so-called disorder 'comprise[s] alternative forms of order, entailing priorities that are perhaps uncomfortable for, or dissonant with, mainstream values' (Fraser and Moore, 2008, p. 748). In short, it recognises that apparently disordered behaviours are equally legitimate responses to an HIV diagnosis and, importantly, ones that, far from being 'unstructured', are structured and ordered in their own right, if on a logic that is suppressed by a neoliberal social order.

To return to the extract from TAC's information pamphlet, the third issue I wish to highlight is the emphasis on '[going] on with your life as best you can' and '[staying] as busy as possible' (Clayden et al., 2013, p. 10). Of course, these injunctions are an attempt to normalise the event of the HIV diagnosis and to impart the message that life carries on. This message is important as it helps to counter the view that an HIV diagnosis constitutes a death sentence (which, as we saw, the TAC itself sometimes iterated in the period pre-ART). However, the accompanying exhortation to 'stay as busy as possible' appears to encourage a kind of mindless busyness that suppresses the emotional response associated with an HIV diagnosis. On this basis, it is possible to argue that the advice, although well-meaning and helpful in some respects, only briefly acknowledges the feelings of shock and fear that might accompany a diagnosis. By recommending activity and distraction as an antidote to negative or troubling emotions, this approach implicitly discourages the newly diagnosed person from engaging in introspection and self-examination. Indeed, the subject position of rational, self-controlled biological citizen seems to encourage the suppression of emotion by instating the (masculine) neoliberal norms of self-control, rationality and proactive planning ('make a plan to get the best care and treatment possible').

The second step in TAC's information booklet is entitled 'Stay connected to your clinic' (Clayden et al., 2013, p. 10). The text below this instruction notes that:

> You may have received information when you learned you were HIV positive, but you may still have a thousand more questions. Be strong and confident about asking everything you are not clear about. For example you may have many questions about passing HIV on to your family or partner. (Clayden et al., 2013, p. 10)

TAC's advice that newly diagnosed individuals seek more information on HIV articulates with the imperatives of informational bio-citizenship, as defined by Rose: it is about each person taking responsibility for her or his health, through the 'active search for scientific knowledge' and the enhancement of their 'biomedical literacy' (Rose, 2007, p. 141). However well-intentioned the injunctions of informational bio-citizenship may be, they operate in this case to place a potentially onerous expectation on the newly diagnosed HIV-positive person to return to the clinic to ask for more HIV-related information soon after diagnosis. Such an expectation may be difficult to meet for people living far from clinics and/or those who are sick at the time of their diagnosis or, indeed, too distressed to confront the news. Moreover, in the case of HIV-positive men, gendered norms associated with health-seeking behaviour may act as a further impediment to actively seeking follow-up advice and care from clinics (Colvin *et al.*, 2010).

In sum, TAC's advice on living with HIV is motivated by a drive to impose regularity and structure on apparent chaos, to schematise, categorise and delimit available responses to an HIV diagnosis. This drive manifests strongly when it comes to the ordering and management of HIV/AIDS because of its association with the unpredictable threats of illness and death. As Waldby cogently observes:

> [t]he spectres of sexual infection, contagion and epidemic arguably present the greatest provocation to this schematising drive. They represent the limit case of its powers in the face of proliferating viral life and the chaos of illness and death, the most profound challenge to the capacities of governance and the maintenance of social order. (Waldby, 1996, p. 141)

The advice that a newly a diagnosed HIV-positive person 'plan and structure' their life can thus be understood as an attempt to contain the threat of HIV, to establish order out of the seeming chaos and uncertainty of illness and to erase the spectre of death surrounding HIV.[4] Insofar as this schematising drive idealises the masculine ideals of rationality, agency and self-control, it involves the repudiation of their presumed feminine opposites: irrationality, passivity and lack of control. Given this gendering of citizenship norms, those considered feminine or feminised because of a symbolic-material association with irrationality, passivity and irresponsibility (for example, women, men who have sex with men, drug users and sex workers) risk being seen as failing to meet the masculine norms of citizenship. Addressing this risk requires a willingness to interrogate the ideals of health citizenship, querying its exclusionary tendencies and finding ways to disrupt its binary logic. In the next chapter, I aim to do just this by challenging the received valuations of agency, responsibility and self-control within contemporary regimes of biopower. I propose a more inclusive, post-humanist understanding of these phenomena – one that challenges their status as being solely the prerogative of individual human subjects.

Conclusion

This chapter has examined two conceptions of the relationship between HIV/AIDS and poverty, both of which, despite their differences, rely on the biological/social dualism: disease as either biological *or* social in origin. The TAC endorsed the biomedical explanation for AIDS arguing that, although poverty contributes to the disease, HIV is most properly understood as a viral infection. It cited lack of access to health care as the reason for the concentration of the South African HIV epidemic among the poor. By contrast, the government understood AIDS as social in origin, arguing that AIDS is a symptom of endemic poverty in South Africa. Both accounts, I argue, prove inadequate in the face of the disease's complexity: AIDS cannot be understood only as a syndrome caused by a virus (a biological object), nor merely as a symptom of social factors such as poverty, which appear resistant to change. By holding fast to the biological/social dualism, these conceptions of disease preclude, or at least limit, the possibility of understanding HIV/AIDS as thoroughly biological and social, its materiality forged through the inextricable entanglements of biological and social forces.

These accounts matter because they not only shape HIV, but also those living with, or dying from, the disease. In this regard, and as the previous discussion highlighted, two quite different enactments of the HIV-positive subject emerge through the government's discourse: they are figured as both victims and vectors of HIV/AIDS. Their status as victims of disease (and poverty) positions them as relatively powerless to prevent infection, while their status as vectors of disease figures them as somehow culpable (and therefore blameworthy) for contracting HIV. Crucially, through their iteration, these ideas shape the very substance of disease, materialising it in specific, sometimes unhelpful ways. For example, where HIV/AIDS is understood as the inevitable consequence of poverty and poor people are presumed to be disease vectors, the measures taken to prevent the spread of HIV reproduce this assumed causal link, thereby undermining attempts to break the symbolic-material association between disease and poverty.

As I have argued, the subject of HIV does not precede social and political forces but rather emerges through them. When these forces change, so too does the subjectivity of those living with HIV. This is perhaps most clearly evident in the marked shift that occurred in TAC's depiction of the HIV-positive subject before and after the introduction of HIV treatment in South Africa. Before ART became publicly available, affected individuals figure in TAC statements as victims of HIV/AIDS and victims of the government's poor policy decisions. By contrast, post-ART they are enlisted as agentive biological citizens in TAC's health promotion literature and, as such, they are encouraged to assume responsibility for managing their health and staving off illness. Because this concept of citizenship idealises the masculine norms of rationality, agency and self-control, it involves the repudiation of their presumed feminine opposites: irrationality, passivity and lack of self-control. Technologies of biological citizenship therefore pose a risk to those HIV-positive subjects viewed as feminine or feminised in some way, including children, men who have sex with men, disabled people, ethnic minorities, drug users and sex workers. By virtue of their presumed irrationality, passivity and intemperance, these already marginalised subjects risk being disqualified from full citizenship. As the analysis in the next chapter reveals, denial of citizenship carries heavy costs for HIV-positive people in terms of their access to rights and protections, including the right to life-saving health care.

In comparing the government and TAC's accounts of the relationship between HIV/AIDS and poverty, this chapter has revealed how, as an effect of the apparent polarisation of the debate, biomedical and social understandings of disease tended to be treated as mutually exclusive. However, it is likely that, beyond the confines of a polarised debate and outside their most heated speeches, both the Mbeki government and TAC would advance a more nuanced, relational conception of HIV causation that recognises the role of both biological and social forces in shaping the disease, its distribution and effects. In other words, I suggest that their views actually share more in common than existing popular and scholarly accounts allow. Extending this point, it is possible to argue that the polarised debate belied any shared ground in TAC's and the government's approaches to HIV, and prevented each party from conceding the legitimacy of the other's position. Moreover, as I have suggested, it is possible to challenge the assumption that the biomedical and the social are ontologically distinct categories and to posit disease as always already a biosocial phenomenon. Indeed, effective, nuanced HIV interventions depend on the ability to understand the biological dimensions of the disease (its presumed underlying nature) as inextricably entangled with the social, cultural and political realities through which it is materialised. Observing the social constructedness of disease is not to imply that disease has no biological reality. Neither is it to downplay the damaging material effects of disease. Rather, it is to draw attention to the (often overlooked) role of social forces in shaping the ontology of disease and its effects. As Singer puts it, in defending what she calls the social origins of disease:

> This is not a denial of the material reality of biology, nor of the real effects of pathogenic agents and other disease causing entities. How we think about their health effects, how we group and label them, the meanings we invest in them, how we act on this construction *(i.e. the making of disease)* is not specified in biology. It is a cultural process. (Singer, 2004, p. 13, original emphasis)

The approach to disease described here invites the recognition that, in the context of South Africa, HIV/AIDS both embodies and helps to (re)produce poverty. I am proposing, in other words, an approach that attends to the ways in which HIV/AIDS and poverty jointly produce ontologies of the disease that are unique to South Africa. This might involve, for example, the design of a treatment policy that aims not only to ensure the successful delivery of ART, but also to redress the persistent social inequalities that shape the distribution, effects and, indeed, the materiality of HIV in South Africa. It could include provisions for some or all of the following:

- monitoring and addressing mismanagement in the public health system (Amado *et al.*, 2012);
- state-subsidised formal housing;
- a universal basic income grant; and
- improving delivery of basic municipal services and infrastructure (Roux and Nyamukachi, 2005), particularly in informal housing settlements and rural areas.

It is encouraging to note that some policies and initiatives are already in place to address some of these issues. Perhaps most significantly, South Africa's current National Strategic Plan (NSP) for HIV includes a set of goals addressing the structural barriers to HIV prevention, care and treatment (Department of Health, 2012). One of these goals directly addresses the poverty–disease nexus by aiming to strengthen poverty reduction and food security programmes. However, despite the NSP's laudable aim of addressing the poverty–HIV dynamic, it is noteworthy that the emphasis is very much on testing and treatment with 85 per cent of the total budget allocated to these programmes (Amado et al., 2012). In terms of the provision of public housing subsidies, the ANC government introduced housing subsidies for low-income households as part of its Reconstruction and Development Program (RDP), and by 2009 75 per cent of South African households were living in formal housing (Shapurjee and Charlton, 2013). Notwithstanding the massive investment in housing and the delivery of almost 3 million houses since 1994, informal housing persists in some areas (Shapurjee and Charlton, 2013).

In relation to the provision of universal basic income support, two South African activist groups, the Khayelitsha Progressive Youth Movement and the New Women's Movement, have held protests demanding a basic income grant (Shapurjee and Charlton, 2013). Yet despite the backing of many civil society organisations and broad popular support (Harris et al., 2011), the South African government has yet to propose basic income support measures. Finally, poor municipal service delivery is a persistent challenge facing the South African government, and service delivery protests and related efforts to improve the delivery of basic municipal services are ongoing (Amado et al., 2012).

As mentioned, it is heartening to see that some measures are already in place to address the HIV–poverty nexus in South Africa, but many challenges remain, not least the lack of basic income support for vulnerable households, and mismanagement in the public health system that undermines the reliable provision of ART (Bateman, 2013). In light of these ongoing challenges and the enduring association of HIV/AIDS and poverty, the policy suggestions above are worth considering. Moreover, while I acknowledge the challenge of affording all the measures proposed here, it is important to stress that pursuing even just one or two of them would change other domains too. If we understand objects as multiply co-constituted phenomena, whatever investments are made in one phenomenon (here HIV/AIDS) will extend to others. That is, the effects of particular responses to disease would be more far-reaching than one can anticipate because HIV/AIDS is, as we have seen, always already entangled with other social problems such as poverty, unemployment, material disadvantage and an uneven distribution of health care.

4
Disease as a Politics of the Human

In Chapters 2 and 3, I demonstrated how the positions of the two major actors in the South African HIV conflict were seemingly polarised. The Treatment Action Campaign's (TAC's) position focused on the patent wrongs of the government position and turned to science to provide the answers to South Africa's growing epidemic. By contrast, Mbeki and his supporters endorsed an AIDS dissident account that emphasised the role of poverty and other so-called social factors in shaping the disease in Africa. Drawing attention to the material effects of the debate's presumed polarisation and to the shared ground it belied, the preceding chapters explored the performative role of binary oppositions – e.g. science/pseudo-science, biology/society, science/politics, agents/victims – in making the disease and its subjects. This chapter continues the deconstructive work of the book by examining another key phenomenon bound up with the politics of HIV in South Africa, the 'human'. It explores the debate's mobilisation of the human/nonhuman binary in terms of how it makes the disease of HIV and its 'human' subjects. Extending the argument made in previous chapters that the government's and TAC's positions were not as starkly split as most reports suggest, I identify another important commonality in their statements on HIV, namely their reliance on a Western liberal humanist conception of the human. I begin by exploring the Mbeki government's resistance to the perceived dehumanisation of Africans in orthodox scientific discourses on HIV and its efforts to include Africans in the liberal humanist category of the human. In its pursuit of an inclusive notion of the human, the Mbeki government relies on a form of anti-colonial, redemptive humanism that resists the Eurocentric values of liberal humanism and develops a racially inclusive notion of the human. While it alters the borders of the human, this inclusive humanism nonetheless leaves intact the human/non-human binary associated with traditional liberal humanism and thus ultimately reinforces the dominance of Western epistemologies and their sometimes unhelpful effects. I then look at the TAC in the same way, demonstrating how its reliance on the discourse of human rights also reproduces a Western liberal humanist view of the human with all the problems it entails.

'We too are human': the assertion of African humanity

In a lengthy essay articulating the government's AIDS dissident position, the authors urge their fellow Africans to:

> stand up to say that we have had enough of the insults that demean Africans, whatever their nationality. The time has come that we gather the courage and the intellect to say that we too are human, as human as any other human being. (Anonymous, 2002, Chapter 15)

As this statement makes clear, the Mbeki government's AIDS dissidence was animated in part by a concern to reassert the humanity of Africans in the wake of centuries of racism and dehumanisation. The importance of valorising African identity is foregrounded in the opening statements of the essay, which stress that 'the war to defeat AIDS is also a war to defeat the humiliation and dehumanisation of the African people' (Anonymous, 2002, Chapter 1). This theme is also evident in the essay's sub-title, 'HIV/AIDS and the Struggle for the Humanisation of the African' and is taken up again more fully in Chapter 11 of the document. The chapter consists of a pastiche of quotations and paraphrases describing the racist stereotypes about African people that allegedly permeate the scientific literature on HIV/AIDS, including that Africans are sexually unrestrained, promiscuous and 'incapable of civilised behaviour' (Chirimuuta and Chirimuuta, 1997, cited in Anonymous, 2002, Chapter 11). It ends with an impassioned denunciation of these stereotypes, through the use of irony:

> Yes, we are sex-crazy! Yes, we are diseased! Yes, we spread the deadly HI Virus through our uncontrolled heterosexual sex! In this regard, yes we are different from the US and Western Europe! Yes, we, the men, abuse women and the girl-child [sic] with gay abandon! Yes, among us rape is endemic because of our culture! Yes, we do believe that sleeping with young virgins will cure us of AIDS! Yes, as a result of all this, we are threatened with destruction by the HIV/AIDS

pandemic! Yes, what we need, and cannot afford, because we are poor, are condoms and anti-retroviral drugs! Help! (Anonymous, 2002, Chapter 11)

The point may be overstated but it reveals that, for the Mbeki government, to concede the scientific orthodoxy on HIV was to resuscitate a racist view of African men as violent and sexually deviant vectors for disease. The Mbeki government's AIDS dissidence can therefore be understood, in part, as an attempt to restore African dignity and humanity by rejecting racist renditions of African masculinity.

This insistence on reaffirming the humanity of African people is, as we know, not an uncommon strategy in anti-colonial struggles.[1] One can hardly disagree with the spirit of this mode of resistance or with the emancipatory logic that the humanity and dignity of African people should be affirmed. Indeed, it is consistent with postcolonial scholar Frantz Fanon's critique of the racism implicit in Western humanism and his articulation of an anti-racist, inclusive humanism or, in his words, a 'new humanism' (Fanon, 1967a, p. 7). It is noteworthy that Fanon is cited twice in the document quoted above, first to endorse claims about the denial of African humanity and, second, in a discussion arguing that Africans' internalised oppression is an effect of colonial domination. In elaborating on 'new humanism', Fanon argued that the ties linking humanism to Eurocentric, racist values could be broken. He therefore called for an emancipatory humanism that 'create[s] the whole man [sic] whom Europe has been incapable of bringing to triumphant birth' (Fanon, 1967b, p. 253).[2]

While acknowledging the value of an anti-colonial, anti-racist strategy that asserts African humanity, it is nevertheless important to consider whether the ties that bind humanism to racism, colonialism, sexism and other forms of domination can be severed. As Diana Fuss (1996, p. 2) stresses in a more recent assessment, the category human is a:

> weapon of potent ideological force, its unstable boundaries perpetually drawn and redrawn to exclude entire groups of socially disempowered groups: the homeless, mothers on welfare, blacks in prison, people with HIV/AIDS, illegal 'aliens'. The human is not, and never has been, an all-inclusive category.

In a similar vein, feminist postcolonial scholar Meyda Yeğenoğlu (1998, p. 95) makes the acute observation that 'the formation of universal humanism's ideal is predicated on a racist gesture, for, in order to be able to proclaim its humanity, the West needed to proclaim its others as slaves and monsters'. In keeping with Yeğenoğlu's point, we can understand the Mbeki government's persistent affirmation of African humanity as an attempt to reclaim 'African-ness' from the realm of the abject Other. But if one accepts that traditional humanism buttresses racism and is a fantasy of singularity and homogeneity, it becomes necessary to consider what is at stake in redrawing the boundaries of the human/non-human to include those abject others who were previously relegated to the domain of the non-human. Or to put this in terms of the Mbeki government's African nationalist discourse we might reasonably ask: what are the unintended ramifications of the government's appeal to a more inclusive humanism? One possible answer is that by defying colonial stereotypes that enact Africans as sub-human and asserting the humanity of Africans, Mbeki actually forces Africans into the Western liberal category of the human. Forcing Africans into an exclusionary Western concept of the human undermines the status of 'African-ness' and runs the risk of reducing the African subject to 'a caricatured imprint of the coloniser's image – as one who cannot be imagined in his own terms, but only in oppositional violence to the latter' (Kumar, 2011, p. 1567). Crucially, this mode of resistance leaves unexamined the notion of the human and its investments in a model of Western humanism that has been complicit with the pernicious practices of colonialism, racism and imperialism (Karavanta and Morgan, 2008). In other words, it leaves unquestioned (and therefore unchanged) the political investments and 'colonizing designs' of the category itself (Fuss, 1996, p. 2).

Extending the feminist critiques above, I argue that a critique of humanism necessitates consideration of whether it is sufficient, or even possible, to reconstitute the notion of the human in ways that are inclusive and de-racialised or whether a more radical move is needed, one that disrupts the status of the human as foundational by challenging the anthropocentrism of humanism. Beyond simply contesting the exclusion of certain groups of people from the domain of the human as Mbeki and his supporters did, such a move would require a more searching treatment of humanism itself, including scrutiny of the ontological and ethical implications of a continued allegiance to humanism (even a more inclusive form of humanism). For example, it might prompt consideration of questions such as the following:

- What exclusions are produced by remaining faithful to an anthropocentric view of the human? In other words, who/what 'is excluded

from mattering' by the reiteration of a Western humanist philosophy (Barad, 2007, p. 235)?
- What differences are homogenised in the human? Here one could argue that HIV in South Africa was a battleground for two key masculinist notions, namely science and nation. As such, and as discussed in Chapter 2, the question of gender tended to be sidelined, erasing the role of violent masculinities and unequal gender relations in producing a feminised HIV epidemic in South Africa.
- How is the human defined in relation to 'nature' or the 'non-human world' and what risks attend the conventional view that humans are 'nature-transcending beings' (Anderson, 2007, p. 199)? For example, how might such a view connect with discourses of human exceptionalism that legitimate oppressive practices against animals as 'non-humans'? How might it encourage a view of the virus as nature, with all the myth making that goes with nature?

These questions, and their implications for the making of HIV in South Africa, are foreclosed by Mbeki's appeal to a more inclusive form of humanism as part of his broader struggle against racism and colonialism. Instead this mode of resistance prematurely reifies the human as the foundational subject within a politics of African nationalism. With this critique in mind, I now turn to a key question animating this book: how does the government's appeal to a more inclusive conception of the 'human' help to materialise HIV as disease?

HIV/AIDS as a threat to the humanity of Africans

In the opening to Chapter 15 of the essay sub-titled 'HIV/AIDS and the Struggle for the Humanisation of the African', the authors state:

> We are poor. We live in conditions of under-development [...] None of this makes us sub-human. Nor should the impact of disease, including AIDS, that afflicts us, be used in the name of *questionable science* and friendship with us, to reduce us to a peculiar species of humanity likely to slip back into a state of savagery. (Anonymous, 2002, Chapter 15, emphasis added)

'Questionable science' on the HIV epidemic in Africa is figured in this statement as a threat to the humanity of Africans. But what constitutes 'questionable science'? As discussed in Chapter 2, the Mbeki executive critiqued what it saw as the racism lodged in orthodox scientific accounts of HIV/AIDS. It claimed that these accounts stereotype black Africans as sexually promiscuous reservoirs of disease, which both harbour and spread infection (Cameron, 2005; Gevisser, 2009). Against this backdrop, we can read 'questionable science', in the government's terms, as racist science. According to Mbeki and his supporters, it reduces African people to 'a state of savagery' and in so doing, denies their humanity (Anonymous, 2002, Chapter 15).

It is perhaps easy to dismiss the government's concerns on the basis that some early scientific accounts of HIV were nothing more than racist misrepresentations of the disease. However, to do so would be to treat racism and science as separate from the disease itself. Indeed, it would be presume that disease has some immutable essence, which is merely misrepresented (but not constituted or changed) by racist science. This book challenges this familiar view of disease, arguing that racist science and its associated disease concepts have shaped the ontology of the disease in Africa. For example, through their iteration, statements that attribute the spread and impact of HIV in Africa to 'sexual promiscuity' produce a causal link between HIV and promiscuity. Public health strategies are then directed at groups presumed to be at increased risk of infection because of their perceived promiscuity – for example, sex workers, migrant workers and Africans. These strategies performatively *constitute* these groups as 'high-risk populations' and, as such, may enable the public perception that they are potentially contagious carriers of HIV. Furthermore, statements linking HIV in Africa to 'promiscuity' reify and naturalise the binary distinctions between the 'West' and 'Africa' and, importantly, between the 'human' subject and 'less than fully human' others. In the process, Africans are depicted (and therefore constituted) as the West's abject Other. They become the 'less than fully human' or 'non-human' against which the human status of the Western subject is defined. These conceptions of disease are powerful because they directly shape the disease and its subjects. To dismiss them as separate from and posterior to the epidemic is to overlook their performative role in producing the epidemic. In short, I am suggesting that we take seriously Mbeki's concerns about how certain conceptualisations of HIV ('questionable science' in his terms) might pose a threat to what he calls African humanity. Reading these concerns through the concept of 'intra-action' illuminates the ways in which HIV and its high prevalence rates in southern Africa, intra-acted with racist assumptions about African sexual difference to produce two mutually constituted phenomena: (1) HIV as a disease of sexual deviance and (2) African subjects as less than fully human. Ironically, as noted in the previous chapter,

Mbeki's resistance to the scientific orthodoxy did little to disrupt these enactments of HIV and its African subjects. If anything, it arguably helped to cement them by entrenching the HIV epidemic and worsening its effects in South Africa. By this I mean that Mbeki's resistance to the scientific orthodoxy meant his government refused to deliver anti-retroviral therapy (ART), and without access to ART, hundreds of thousands of South Africans died from AIDS.

Where the impact of HIV is seen as an existential threat to African humanity, one response is to deny the severity of the threat, as Mbeki and his supporters did. They contested established estimates of HIV prevalence, incidence and mortality in South Africa, and argued that diseases of poverty, not HIV/AIDS, constitute the biggest national problem:

> *It* [a document describing the government's AIDS dissident position] *rejects* as baseless and self-serving the assertion that millions of our people are HIV positive [...]
>
> *It rejects* the assertion that, among the nations, we have the highest incidence of HIV infection and AIDS deaths, caused by sexual immorality among our people.
>
> *It rejects* the claim that AIDS is the single largest cause of death in our country [...]
>
> *It rejects* the argument to 'break the silence' about AIDS by imposing the silence of the grave about diseases of poverty. (Anonymous, 2002, preface, original emphasis)

Although the Mbeki government did not consistently reject accepted HIV estimates, it often claimed that they were inflated, citing statistics from alternative and usually outdated sources to support the argument that 'South Africa falls significantly below the average for the African countries with the lowest incidence of AIDS' (Anonymous, 2002, preface). Crucially, alternative HIV prevalence and incidence statistics do not simply *represent* the impact of the disease differently. Rather, they are part of the epidemiological apparatus that *materialises* disease and, in this case, that materialises it in ways that challenge the scientific orthodoxy.

One of the early scientific accounts of HIV/AIDS provides a striking example of the performative power of epidemiology to make disease in specific, sometimes unhelpful ways. Some first-wave epidemiological studies converged with popular prejudice to conceive HIV as a gay disease, naming it gay related immune deficiency disease (GRID). In an analysis of the changing epidemiological understanding of HIV, Oppenheimer draws attention to the role of what he calls the 'epidemiological imagination' in figuring HIV as a 'gay disease' when it was first named in the early 1980s:

> Given their training, epidemiologists fairly consistently defined HIV infection as a biological process occurring within a determinate social matrix. That the infection was first identified among young male homosexuals and intravenous drug users certainly reinforced this professional proclivity. The results of this exercise in epidemiological imagination were complex and equivocal [...] the epidemiologists' approach may have skewed the choice of models and hypotheses, determined which data were excluded from consideration until later in the epidemic, and offered scientific justification for popular prejudice, particularly against gay men. (Oppenheimer, 1988, p. 268)

Oppenheimer's reference to the 'exercise in epidemiological imagination' captures very effectively the point that epidemiological data, like all scientific data, are always already political; they are part of the politics that makes disease. Epidemiology directs services, which then impact on rates of infection and mortality, thus materially shaping disease and, in turn, epidemics.

With this in mind, let us consider the implications of the government's use of epidemiological data showing South Africa's incidence rate as significantly lower than that of other African countries. It is possible to see this as an attempt by the government to contain the perceived threat that the HIV epidemic posed to the human status of Africans. However, the government also contributed to constituting the disease differently: contrary to conventional epidemiological accounts which characterise HIV in South Africa as a high prevalence epidemic, it cited epidemiological data suggesting a lower prevalence rate (as compared to other sub-Saharan African countries). This enabled the government to minimise the problem and adjust its policy response accordingly. By arguing that HIV is a relatively low prevalence epidemic, symptomatic of a larger problem of endemic poverty, Mbeki and his supporters could justify the government's limited public health spending on HIV and its policy focus on poverty alleviation strategies. Public health experts and opposition parties have criticised the Mbeki government's expenditure on HIV. They maintain that it was an insufficient response to the epidemic, enabling HIV to spread and thus making the epidemic in South Africa more severe (Hartley, 2001). Extending this criticism, it is possible to argue that, by minimising the problem of HIV and prioritising other social problems (notably poverty), the Mbeki government allowed resources to be redirected away from HIV. This meant that access to HIV screening, prevention and treatment would have declined, or at least not kept pace with South Africa's growing epidemic. In Barad's terms, we can say that the government's AIDS dissidence intra-acted with a presumption of a relatively low HIV prevalence rate, a reduced HIV/AIDS budget, the decision not to deliver ART, and inadequate HIV prevention measures to help produce at least three damaging effects: (1) more HIV infections, (2) higher numbers of preventable AIDS-related deaths and (3) a materially altered epidemic, one which was more severe than it might otherwise have been.

As this example reveals, disease incidence and prevalence rates matter because they shape the view of the policy problem requiring a response, which in turn affects the range and scale of public health measures taken to address it. The point is that these phenomena do not simply *represent* or *respond* to an apparently self-evident, stable disease; rather they jointly help to *materialise* the disease, its distribution and effects. Therefore, the political conflict over HIV, including the contestation over which statistical data 'accurately reflect' the epidemiology of the disease and the data themselves have all contributed to the materiality of HIV in South Africa, yet these factors are typically considered irrelevant to the apparently self-evident 'facts' of the disease. Treating political conflict and discursive practices (epidemiology, policy and so on) as intra-active elements of disease in the making enables us to convert disease from a 'matter of fact' to a 'matter of concern': an emergent phenomenon forged through (rather than preceding) politics.

The struggle for HIV treatment: mobilising human rights

The Mbeki government was not solely responsible for rendering HIV a disease of the human; the concept of the 'human' was equally central to TAC's position, although it was mobilised differently to fight for treatment access, rather than to valorise African identity. The TAC framed their battle for universal, free HIV treatment as a rights-based movement, arguing that access to treatment was a *human* right, protected by the South African constitutional guarantee of equal access to health care services. As I will demonstrate, TAC's reliance on humanism, as part of its human rights discourse, also has implications for how HIV and those affected by it (its 'human' subjects) are differentially constituted.

In 2001, the TAC filed a lawsuit against the government, contending that the state's failure to develop a comprehensive programme for prevention of mother-to-child transmission (PMTCT) of HIV violated constitutional provisions regarding the (human) rights to life, equality, dignity, and bodily and psychological integrity:

> the State has ensured that efficacious drugs for the prevention of HIV infection are placed beyond the reach of most people in this country. This constitutes a profound threat to the fundamental rights of South Africans to:
>
> - access to health care services, including reproductive health care (section 27);
> - basic health care services for children (section 28(1)(c));
> - life (section 11);
> - human dignity (section 10);
> - equality (section 9); and
> - psychological integrity, including the right to make decisions regarding reproduction (section 12(2)(a)). (Marcus and Majola, 2001, para. 1.11.4)

In their pleadings, the TAC and its co-applicants also argued that the government's PMTCT policy violated the South African Bill of Rights:

> Section 7(3) of the Constitution places a duty on the State to 'respect, protect, promote and fulfil the rights in the Bill of Rights'. Section 237 of the Constitution requires that 'all constitutional obligations must be performed diligently and without delay'.
>
> The policy adopted by the respondents in selectively making Nevirapine available only at designated sites is not only unreasonable, arbitrary and irrational, but creates an untenable inequality which discriminates against the poor [...] [The TAC] acts in the public interest in ensuring the effective enforcement of the constitutional rights that are at issue in this matter. (Marcus and Majola, 2001, paras 1.11.2–1.11.3, 2.2.4)

These statements exemplify how the legal struggle for PMTCT services was fought and won on the grounds of human rights with South Africa's High Court ruling that the prohibition of the 'use of Nevirapine outside the pilot sites in the public health sector [was...] an unjustifiable barrier to the progressive realization of the *right to health care*' (TAC, 2001, p. 31, emphasis added).[3] Although not dismissing the importance of the TAC case for successfully holding the state to its constitutional duty of care, I wish to question the notion of the 'universal human' on which the case relies. Who is the privileged subject of human rights? Is this subject as inclusive as appeals to universal human rights would have us believe? Feminists have argued that, because rights-based approaches are oriented to heterosexual, masculinist ideals and instate the European male subject as the 'universal, prototypical human', they support male, heterosexual privilege (Otto, 1997, p. 5). Postcolonial scholars, meanwhile, have pointed out the ways in which claims to the universality of human rights have serviced the 'disciplinary civilizing mission of Europe' by denying rights to indigenous people (Otto, 1997, p. 5). Both strands of critique challenge the proclaimed universality of human rights by exposing how the 'human' of rights discourse is narrowly defined to exclude the majority of people, thereby protecting a white, Western male minority. This is not to suggest that rights cannot be used to emancipate people. As the TAC case illustrates, they certainly can and have been used successfully as emancipatory tools to win small gains for marginalised groups. But because they rely on the problematic of the human (defined against the non-human), rights claims always produce a series of inclusions and exclusions: they work to emancipate particular subjects, but simultaneously discipline and exclude others from the dominant social order. Struggles fought on the shifting terrain of human rights do little to challenge the exclusionary logic of humanism. They simply extend the borders of the rights-bearing, human subject and inevitably produce further exclusions in the form of a different set of 'less than fully human' Others.

Returning to the contemporary context, some evidence suggests that this exclusionary logic plays out in the South African public health care system to produce treatment inequalities between South African citizens and non-citizens. Although the right to health care is, in principle, accorded to 'all persons' in South Africa, recent reports suggest that, in practice, Mozambican, Zimbabwean and Lesotho nationals seeking treatment in the public health system are sometimes subjected to substandard care or even denied HIV treatment on the basis of their foreign nationality (Amon and Todrys, 2009; Crush and Tawodzera, 2011). It would appear that, despite South Africa's progressive Bill of Rights, the right to health care is seen in some public institutions as dependent on prior citizenship status, leading to claims that migrants are subjected to 'medical xenophobia' (Human Rights Watch, 2008, p. 1). Following feminist critiques of human rights, it is possible to argue that, as non-citizens, migrants are effectively constituted as lesser humans and are thus perceived by some public health officials as having fewer (or no) rights to access social services, including health care. To elaborate further on the exclusions that accompany rights claims in the context of HIV in South Africa, the next section explores the connections between TAC's rights-based struggle for HIV treatment and its promotion of biological citizenship in the post-treatment era. It considers the norms that biological citizenship instates and how they can operate to allow some subjects to qualify as citizens and to disqualify others from full citizenship. It also explores what might happen to those who fail to qualify as rights-bearing health citizens. These issues extend beyond the matter of whether all HIV-positive people in South Africa are equally entitled to rights. They have implications for how individuals and communities are themselves produced by claims to human rights and, by extension, conferrals of citizenship. They are worth addressing because, as we know, not everyone is entitled to citizenship and thus to access the rights and protections associated with it.

Treatment in the making of biological citizens

As discussed in Chapter 3, the implementation of a comprehensive ART programme in South Africa enabled a shift in TAC's activism towards ensuring the successful delivery of HIV treatment and promoting treatment literacy and adherence. The success of ART is depicted in public health discourse as contingent on a model of responsibilised citizenship, in which patients take individual responsibility for adhering to strict treatment regimes, thus removing the need for external surveillance models of treatment such as Directly Observed Therapy for Tuberculosis (DOT-TB) (Robins, 2006). Over and above the demands of treatment adherence, the discourses of health citizenship place imperatives on HIV-positive subjects to disclose their HIV status, abstain from heavy drinking and smoking, practise safe sex and maintain a healthy diet. TAC's approach to monitoring treatment delivery and promoting adherence conforms closely to this model of health citizenship: in TAC's health promotion literature, HIV-positive subjects are enlisted as what Rose (2007) would call 'biological citizens' who take individual responsibility for their health. 'Healthy living' is promoted using the discourse of empowerment as the route to personal 'fulfilment' and 'freedom' (Rose, 2007). Furthermore, the ideals of patient empowerment, choice and self-determination are often construed as 'rights' (Petersen *et al.*, 2010). For example, according to the South African Bill of Rights, everyone has the right to 'access to health care services, including reproductive health care' (Republic of South Africa, 1996, section 27). It was precisely this right to health care that the TAC enforced in relation to the provision of PMTCT.

The TAC has continued to invoke this rights-based discourse since ART was introduced. For example, in a health promotion pamphlet on 'living with HIV', it cites South Africa's Patient Rights Charter to remind HIV-positive patients of their rights:

> Having HIV does not make you a second-class citizen. You have a right to confidentiality: it is the law. Clinics are not allowed to discriminate against you. Our government has issued a Patients' Rights Charter that says: 'Everyone has the right to access to health care services that include provision for special needs in case of [...] a person living with HIV or AIDS patients'. Unfortunately, some healthcare workers still do not comply with the charter. Later in this handbook we give you some suggestions of what you can do if this happens. (Clayden et al., 2013, p. 11)

In later sections on 'Attending the Clinic' and 'Support Groups', the TAC handbook elaborates on how HIV-positive people can enforce their right to health care by offering the following advice:

> Ask the nurse or doctor what he or she finds when examining you. Ask about all results from special tests (X-rays, blood tests). Ask about your medicines and remember their names. If your nurse or doctor does not answer your questions, explain that it is your right to know [...] We have to ensure that our rights are respected. (Clayden et al., 2013, pp. 88–9)

As these statements reveal, TAC's rights-based movement for equal treatment is consistent with neoliberal democratic ideals of individual rights, empowerment and agency: all concepts that are central to the prevailing model of biological citizenship. However, the focus on rights, empowerment and agency obscures the reciprocal responsibilities and obligations of contemporary forms of biological citizenship (Petersen et al., 2010). This makes it necessary to reflect critically on who is being empowered (and, by extension, who is disempowered) by the emphasis on individual rights and apparently unconstrained agency.

If we consider the example cited above, in which individual patients are encouraged to challenge potential infringements on their rights, it is worth asking: to what extent are foreign nationals living with HIV (who may not speak a local language and who may be undocumented migrants fearing deportation) able to enforce their right to HIV treatment?[4] My intention in raising this question is not to diminish the value of TAC's treatment movement and its empowerment of certain HIV-positive collectivities through the mobilisation of new forms of health citizenship. Rather, it is to highlight the need for consideration of the limits of biological citizenship and its implications for those who fail to qualify as rights-bearing citizens. To address this concern, it is instructive to explore the attributes of the biological citizen as they are revealed in an analysis of TAC's health promotion literature. Below is an extract from TAC's handbook on living with HIV. Like the extracts analysed in Chapter 3, it offers advice on how to cope in the first week after an HIV diagnosis:

Step 5: Stay healthy.

Live as healthily as possible! Eat nutritious food and try to exercise. Limit the amount of alcohol you drink and do not smoke. Make sure you monitor your CD4 count regularly and start anti-retroviral treatment (ART) as soon as you need it. (Clayden *et al.*, 2013, p. 11)

This extract exhorts newly diagnosed HIV-positive subjects to manage their health and practise self-care by eating a nutritious diet, continually monitoring their CD4 count, exercising, and avoiding alcohol and smoking. Implicit here is the assumption that managing one's health through ongoing self-surveillance constitutes a reasonable, rational response to being diagnosed with HIV. TAC's emphasis on continual self-care, self-surveillance and health optimisation is also evident in its information sheet entitled 'Monitoring and managing HIV', published in its handbook:

It is important to understand that HIV is a chronic, lifetime condition [...] It is important for you to recognise signs and symptoms – clues that your body gives to tell that you are sick. You should report anything that feels new or different in your body to your doctor. (Clayden *et al.*, 2013, p. 27)

Here the onus to continually monitor health and stave off AIDS-related illness is placed on the HIV-positive subject. If anything, the availability of ART has helped to increase the emphasis on individual self-surveillance as it requires those on treatment to survey their health constantly in order to ensure their viral load remains 'undetectable' (Race, 2001).

These extracts illuminate how TAC's health promotion literature enlists HIV-positive subjects as reasonable, rational and autonomous biological citizens who take individual responsibility for their health. The contemporary health citizen is thus produced as a site of reason, rationality and autonomous will, aligning it with the liberal humanist figure of the human. Because biological citizenship is continually performed, status as a full biological citizen is always in jeopardy. It is always predicated on the pursuit of 'health', 'undetectable viral load' and so on. Therefore, everyone faces potential expulsion from the realm of the citizen, although for some the threat of expulsion is more acute. Keeping this in mind, the question arises: who can escape detection for a less-than-perfect performance of biological citizenship? And, conversely, who might easily be detected and disqualified from full citizenship on the basis that they cannot consistently meet the norms of the contemporary neoliberal health subject? Given that the ideals of biological citizenship – autonomy, reason and rationality – correlate with those of liberal humanism, I suggest that all those historically considered lesser human beings within the Western humanist paradigm risk being disqualified from full citizenship. These 'less than fully' biological citizens might include prisoners, lesbian, gay, bisexual, transgender and intersex (LGBTI) people, sex workers, homeless people, drug users, and undocumented migrants – in short, the most disadvantaged and marginalised subjects. These subjects risk being seen as even more inept citizens – and, by implication, 'inept at being human' (Bauman, 2003, p. 128) – for purportedly failing to follow the injunctions of responsibilised biological citizenship. As Decoteau (2013, p. 149) notes in an analysis of biological citizenship in the context of South Africa, these modes of citizenship, with their emphasis on individual responsibility have 'redefined the contours of exclusion [...] where those on the margins simply fall off the edges of the social because their grasp on the body politic is so tenuous and provisional'. The issue of exclusion from citizenship has particular resonance in South Africa where, until 19 years ago, the black majority was treated as second-class citizens under apartheid. Despite the rights and protections afforded by South Africa's new constitution, the majority of South Africans are, in effect, still less than full citizens by virtue of endemic poverty, social marginalisation and political disenfranchisement. Highlighting this point, Robins and von Lieres (2004, p. 576) observe:

While the legal status of the majority of people [in South Africa] is assured, their experience of citizenship is ambiguous. They often remain excluded from effective economic and political participation. If South Africa's new democracy speaks to anything, it is to the uneasy intertwining of democracy and marginalization.

Given that this legacy of material disadvantage and socio-political marginalisation affects a significant proportion of South Africa's population, it seems unlikely that enforcing the right to health care will enable marginalised communities to claim full (biological) citizenship.

Making live and letting die: biological citizenship in the making of HIV/AIDS

By constituting HIV-positive subjects as unfettered agents who are responsible for their illness, contemporary regimes of biological citizenship can preclude scrutiny of the material effects of public health itself, that is, the ways in which public health discourses (including those associated with biological citizenship) help to constitute the subjects of health, allowing only some to qualify as full biological citizens, and relegating already marginalised others to the domain of failed citizens. This differential enactment of HIV-positive subjects has important ramifications for the prognosis of affected individuals in that it shapes access to health care and life-prolonging treatment. Significantly, then, the enactment of HIV-positive people as either successful biological citizens or failed citizens is active in producing at least two mutually constituted enactments of HIV/AIDS:

1. a chronic, manageable infection – HIV – for those who qualify as (fully human) biological citizens and can access the benefits of citizenship, notably health care;
2. a fatal, debilitating disease – AIDS – for those disqualified from full citizenship and therefore denied the human rights that attend citizenship status, notably the right to health care.

As with other chronic illnesses, these two ontologies of HIV/AIDS also coincide with different stages of disease progression. However, the introduction of ART has enabled HIV and AIDS to be decoupled, challenging the idea of a linear progression from HIV to AIDS. The point here is that the materiality of HIV/AIDS (including its presumed 'progression') is not given in nature and immutable, but rather is socially constituted, produced through social practices and norms, including those associated with the dynamics of citizenship.

If one accepts that contemporary regimes of health citizenship are necessarily exclusionary (because of their reliance on the ideals of liberal humanism), what does this mean for the growing emphasis on biological citizenship as part of the biomedical management of HIV in South Africa and indeed in many liberal democracies across the world? Should biological citizenship be eschewed because of its reliance on the flawed and exclusionary logic of humanism or can it be reconfigured to militate against the risk of excluding already marginalised subjects? Raising these questions is not to advocate that biological citizenship be abandoned, but rather to caution against an uncritical endorsement of its imperatives to reason, responsibility, self-surveillance and individual autonomy. There is cause to consider how these imperatives contribute to the differential constitution of health subjects, allowing a privileged few to qualify as (fully human) rights-bearing citizens, and rendering the most marginalised subjects lesser humans with limited, if any, rights. These marginalised others could all too easily become the casualties of biological citizenship, left to die because of their perceived failure to consistently meet the requirements of citizenship and access the rights attendant on it (Biehl, 2004, 2007; Decoteau, 2013). To put it plainly, attributions of citizenship (and by implication, humanity) matter because they bear directly on biopolitical norms governing who is made to live and who is left to die (Foucault, 2003).

In concluding an analysis of the limits of biological citizenship in a different context – that affecting hepatitis C-positive people who inject drugs – Fraser and Seear stress the need to interrogate the agency and responsibilities of public health itself:

> Hepatitis C-positive people who inject drugs are constantly invited to navigate Kant's three questions [What can I know? What must I do? What may I hope?] to engage, in the process, in a complex and demanding relationship with themselves. But there is a corresponding need to turn these questions around and apply them to medicine and public health as well, and likewise expect them to engage in a relationship with themselves and their ambitions. What can *they* know? What must *they* do? What may *they* hope? If contemporary society has transformed health into a key resource for social and political belonging, medicine and public health's responsibilities for the

most marginalised and disadvantaged are even more substantial than conceived to date. (Fraser and Seear, 2011, p. 108, original emphasis)

In addition to critically examining public health and shifting the focus away from questions of individual agency, it would be helpful to rethink received notions of agency, responsibility and rationality. Rather than figuring these as attributes of individual human subjects, they might usefully be understood as phenomena produced in the encounters of 'humans' and 'non-humans' (however they are defined). On this rethinking, the ideals of biological citizenship, while not equally accessible to all health subjects, are also not simply the outcome of human acts of will. Therefore, those who conform to the imperatives of health citizenship are not better citizens (and, by extension, more superior humans) because they 'possess' the right attributes. In other words, the human subject is not exclusively responsible for whether and how s/he engages the imperatives of biological citizenship. It is necessary to consider the relational field within which 'responsibility', 'agency', 'autonomy' and 'rationality' are produced. HIV-positive subjects undoubtedly play an important role within this field, but they cannot be isolated from it. Instead, the HIV-positive subject and the injunctions of biological citizenship (towards responsibility, agency and so on) are constituted in relation to each other. They are also constituted in relation to the virus, ART, drug shortages, drug side-effects, food security and poverty – to name just a few 'non-human' phenomena that participate in the relational field of HIV.

This point about distributed responsibility and its implications for biological citizenship can usefully be elaborated through reference to three TAC statements on ART adherence. The first two below are excerpted from a TAC treatment literacy booklet titled *ARVs in Our Lives*:

- The challenge to stay on treatment rests with the individual and his or her support structures.
- You have to follow your regimen every day. This includes over the weekend, and in the different situations involved in life. Taking days off your regimen is a very dangerous way of using treatment. There are always things that can help you to avoid missing doses, whatever your lifestyle. (TAC contributors, 2006, preface)

Treatment adherence is presented here as the exclusive responsibility of 'individual' patients and their 'support structures', which are glossed in the TAC booklet as family and community support systems (TAC contributors, 2006, preface). Missed doses are ascribed to the patient's 'lifestyle' and s/he is strongly cautioned against interrupting the regimen on the basis that doing so is a 'very dangerous way of using treatment'. Here, adherence is treated as a 'uniquely "human" [...] responsibility', bracketing out the role of non-human participants, such as poor drug design and treatment efficacy in shaping adherence (Race, 2012, p. 36).

However, a recent TAC statement on drug shortages suggests that problems with ART adherence are not attributable to human frailty alone and that, in fact, there are *not* 'always things that can help [... patients] to avoid missing doses' (TAC contributors, 2006, preface).

> [T]he Treatment Action Campaign (TAC) [and others...] are deeply concerned by widespread stock outs at health facilities in the Eastern Cape, which have been caused by the collapse of the medicines supply chain from the Mthatha Medical Depot [...] The unavailability of these [ARV] medicines is having and will continue to have severe consequences for patients on ART and will result in many developing resistance to their current treatment and others becoming increasingly ill [...] the facility has been dysfunctional and corrupt for several years now [...] Recently, this problem has been exacerbated by the fact that since 10 October 2012, the distribution of medicines from the depot to facilities has been severely compromised by strike action and staff participating in go-slows. (TAC writer, 2012)

Contrary to the advice given in TAC's treatment booklet, it is clear from the above account that ART adherence cannot be seen as the sole responsibility of the human subject. Instead, ART adherence is revealed in this passage as contingent on a complex network of differentially constituted 'human' and 'non-human' forces, including drug shortages, a collapsed medicine supply chain, corrupt public health officials, industrial action, and a dysfunctional public health system. All these phenomena have a part to play and a responsibility to bear in materialising ART adherence, and in producing drug-resistant strains of the virus.

I am not implying that the authors of the TAC booklet are not aware of the factors that powerfully impact the attainability of health and treatment success. Indeed the statement on drug shortages suggests that TAC is seeking to raise awareness of these factors in an effort to improve conditions in the public health system. However, despite these efforts, in some of the appeals to individual responsibility, self-care and so on these other factors drop out of view, in favour of a rather simplistic view that attributes responsibility for treatment adherence to individual subjects. In other words, in the context of health promotion, self-management is foregrounded to the exclusion of other factors that powerfully impact on treatment success. Employing a distributed notion of responsibility could help health promotion discourses to avoid concentrating responsibility unfairly in individual subjects. For example, TAC's advice could be framed to acknowledge that many factors impact on treatment success, including some that are outside the control of individual actors. This acknowledgement does not absolve the HIV-positive subject of responsibility for managing treatment but it recognises that it is not their responsibility alone. I am suggesting here that recommendations that HIV-positive individuals adhere to treatment are accompanied by realistic assessments of the difficulties some may face in doing so and, importantly, by an account of the role of other responsible actors (e.g. public health officials, drug supply chain managers) in facilitating, or impeding, treatment adherence.

Seeing responsibility for adherence as distributed enables an understanding of treatment that avoids attributions of blame, such as the following, which was cited in the TAC booklet as a reason why treatments do not always work: '[P]eople continue to make the same mistakes and move to a new [ARV] combination without understanding why the original one failed' (TAC contributors, 2006, p. 51). Ascribing treatment failure to the 'mistakes' 'people continue to make' precludes the possibility that the design of the treatment itself, with its potentially debilitating side-effects and strenuous adherence requirements, fails patients (TAC contributors, 2006, p. 51). Attributions of patient fallibility are part of the moralising discourse of non-compliance, which works to responsibilise and discipline patients for the unintended effects of biomedical technologies such as ARV drugs (Rosengarten, 2009). Moreover, such attributions presume a liberal humanist view of the wilful, fully conscious subject who takes responsibility (or not) for his/her actions and bears the consequences accordingly.

The point here is to draw attention to the need for scrutiny of the ways in which biological citizenship, with its injunctions towards reason, individual agency and responsibility, risks disqualifying marginalised and disadvantaged subjects from full citizenship. As we have seen, when the model of biological citizenship is applied to managing HIV, it can help to produce two quite different ontologies of disease: a chronic manageable illness (HIV) for those who qualify as (fully human) biological citizens and a life-threatening, terminal illness (AIDS) for those who are deemed failed citizens and lesser humans. These ontologies are implicated in whether affected individuals live with HIV or die prematurely from treatable AIDS-related illnesses. It is the poorest, most marginalised individuals who are likely to be seen as failed biological citizens and there is a risk that, for them, HIV will remain a life-threatening illness, despite treatment being available in principle. Mbeki's appeal to the poverty explanation for HIV is relevant here in that poverty, HIV and social-material disadvantage are revealed as co-constituted. HIV both embodies and helps to (re)produce poverty and disadvantage. Yet discourses of biological citizenship, with their emphasis on individual agency and responsibility, tend to overlook the important role of so-called structural forces (including poverty) in shaping disease and, by extension, limiting the capacity of individuals to meet the obligations of biological citizenship and access its rewards. The neglect of such factors as poverty in materialising disease, and the associated tendency to attribute responsibility for disease to individuals, is one of the limitations of biological citizenship, one that can help to entrench the poverty–disease dynamic.

Conclusion

As we have seen, the government and TAC deployed liberal humanism in quite different ways. The government pursued a redemptive humanism, which, despite its racial inclusiveness, forced Africans into the existing Western liberal category of the human. The TAC, meanwhile, appealed to human rights in its fight for HIV treatment, arguing that the government's HIV policy infringed the (human) rights to life, equality, dignity, and bodily integrity. Despite the seemingly agonistic positions of TAC and the government, and the different ends to which they deployed liberal humanism, they both enacted HIV as a politics of the human. This enactment enabled a homogenisation of differences in the human. The government's pursuit of a redemptive, racially inclusive humanism meant that, as noted in Chapter 2, it foregrounded the question of race and neglected that of gender, specifically the role of violent masculinities and unequal gender relations in producing a feminised HIV epidemic in South Africa. Similarly, by invoking the supposedly universal human of rights discourse, the TAC tended to overlook the performative role of race, socioeconomic status, gender, citizenship and other dimensions of 'human' difference in shaping the substance of HIV, its distribution and effects. In sum, by appealing to an apparently universal human, both parties helped to obscure important differences in terms of gender, race, age, nationality and socioeconomic status in the making of HIV in South Africa. Furthermore, by treating the human as self-evident, the TAC and the government displaced from view the ways in which statements of 'human-ness' produce the 'more and less human', the 'failed human' and the 'non-human'. I am, of course, not suggesting that they did so intentionally (or even consistently) but rather that this was one of the unanticipated and unhelpful effects of their allegiance to a liberal humanist view of the human.

In the case of TAC and its appeals to contemporary modes of biological citizenship, we have seen how the individualising and responsibilising norms of biological citizenship would seem to disqualify socially and materially marginalised HIV-positive subjects from full citizenship. In Rose's (2007, p. 147) terms, these already disadvantaged subjects are produced as 'problematic persons' and risk exclusion from the 'community of responsible biological citizens'. Far from being immaterial, conferrals and denials of citizenship have significant material implications for HIV and its subjects in that they help to produce two qualitatively different (yet co-constituted) ontologies of disease: (1) a chronic manageable illness – HIV – for those who qualify as biological citizens and can access the right to life-saving treatment; (2) a debilitating, terminal illness – AIDS – for those who fail to enact the attributes of individual responsibility and autonomy associated with biological citizenship. For the latter group, the benefits of HIV treatment may remain elusive, if they are available at all. The need to examine the constitutive exclusions of contemporary forms of biopower is perhaps most pressing in post-apartheid South Africa, where experiences of citizenship are still fraught, after a long, unique history of massive exclusion from citizenship. Indeed, despite the official extension of citizenship to black South Africans, civil rights and protections remain 'a far-off dream' for the black majority (Ramphele, 2001, p. 4). In the context of South Africa then, this raises the question of whether the potential inequalities in the formulation of biological citizenship could extend racial inequalities created under apartheid.

Given the potential of biological citizenship to further exclude already marginalised individuals from the realm of the 'proper' neoliberal subject, it would be helpful to rethink its ideals of individual responsibility and unfettered agency. Instead of seeing responsibility and agency as attributes of individual human subjects, I have suggested they could usefully be understood as distributed phenomena, produced in the encounters of humans and non-humans. This extended account of responsibility (and agency) has the potential to change the health promotion approach of organisations such as the TAC. For one, instead of attributing poor adherence to human fallibility, it could mean acknowledging the non-human forces that shape adherence and offering advice on how to deal with them. Exceeding what are usually termed 'structural' forces, non-human forces designate the range of social, cultural and techno-scientific processes that help to constitute realities. In the context of HIV, they include the design of treatment itself, reliable access to drugs, the operation of medical supply chains and the management of the public health system. An extended notion of agency also invites a more reflexive public health approach, one that questions the adequacy of existing treatment technologies and attends to the ways in which they might be said to 'fail patients', rather than the other way round. Such an approach could involve campaigning for improvements in drug design, based on the recognition that the debilitating side-effects and onerous dosing regimens of existing ARV drugs can undermine adherence (Rosengarten, 2009). In short, a distributed notion of responsibility prompts the recognition that individual human subjects are not exclusively responsible for whether and how they conform to the norms of health citizenship. It invites – or perhaps even requires – us to acknowledge that the achievement of citizenship status is contingent on a complex network of human and non-human forces. Doing so may enable us to forge different, more generous forms of biological citizenship, whose ideals and rewards are measured in terms of whether they are accessible to the poorest and most marginalised, who might otherwise be consigned to the fringes of the public health system where life is precarious and death a distinct threat.

To draw these threads together, the analysis conducted in this chapter has elaborated on the book's argument that politics helps to produce disease and its (human) subjects. In the case of the latter, we have seen that politics helps to constitute the subjects of HIV as 'more or less human', 'inept at being human' or 'yet to be humanised' (Bauman, 2003, p. 128). The question of the human (and the ways in which it is variously constituted) also pertains to disease. HIV is not reducible to the status of a non-human object. Neither is it simply an object of science, nor indeed the predictable outcome of political forces. Far exceeding both these conceptions, HIV is perhaps best understood as an emergent phenomenon, made and remade in the dizzying array of intra-actions of humans and non-humans, science and politics, nature and culture. Crucially, HIV is open to change: different intra-actions will produce the disease differently. The recognition of the open-endedness of disease guides the book's concluding chapter as it offers some suggestions for how HIV might be remade in ways that are more compassionate, generous and accountable to those living with the disease, and for all of us who are necessarily entangled with it.

Conclusion: Towards an Ontological Politics of Disease

The field of HIV/AIDS has changed dramatically since the development of anti-retroviral therapy (ART). Yet despite the important contribution of ART, HIV/AIDS remains a very challenging disease to treat, partly because its treatment is fraught with issues of adherence, debilitating side-effects and viral resistance. As I have argued, anti-retroviral (ARV) drugs themselves are productive in that they not only treat HIV (by slowing down viral replication), but can also produce viral mutations. In the process, ARVs too are transformed, rendered less effective or even ineffective in combating the new drug-resistant forms of the virus. As more drug-resistant forms of HIV emerge, the range of available treatment combinations is reduced, making HIV more difficult to treat, and in turn requiring new drugs. Importantly, from the perspective of this book, the phenomena of viral mutations and drug resistance reveal the contingent and emergent nature of the virus, even as it is understood by realist science. The process of viral mutation illuminates the ways in which the virus, HIV treatment and the HIV-positive subject are materialised in their dynamic relations to each other and in relation to other phenomena such as individual rates of adherence, drug side-effects and viral load counts. This book has mapped some of these relations as they play out in one of the most severe HIV epidemics in the world, the South African epidemic. It has traced some of the ontologies of HIV that have emerged in that country, with a special emphasis on tracking the generative role of political contestation in producing forms of the disease that are unique to South Africa. Focusing in particular on the contestation that developed under Mbeki's AIDS dissident government, it explored the negotiations and struggles between the Mbeki executive and civil society organisation Treatment Action Campaign (TAC) over the causes and treatment of HIV. In doing so, the book has attempted to produce a new account of the TAC–government debate, one that moves beyond approaches that foreground only the debate's apparent polarisation by attending instead to important points of continuity across the positions of the key actors. Perhaps most critically, it has also sought to demonstrate how the debate itself (and its perceived polarisation) is part of the politics that makes HIV as disease.

In thinking about how the very materiality of HIV in South Africa has been altered by political struggles and contestation, I was drawn to theoretical-methodological tools that engage the question of matter without assuming *either* that it exists prior to discourse as a fact of nature *or* that it is largely a product of discourse and thus lacks any agency. The work of Bruno Latour proved of especial value in this regard as it takes matter seriously and thus advances a kind of renewed empiricism, but one that avoids retreating into biological determinism and thus reducing matter to the effect of a prematurely reified biology. Latour's expressed unease with some social critiques of fact led him to draw an analytically useful distinction between 'matters of fact' and 'matters of concern'. Instead of trying to destabilise matters of fact and expose them as entirely constructed, Latour proposes a shift in analytic focus to 'matters of concern'. Such a shift does not dispense with facts but rather is concerned to trace their complex history. Challenging the foundational status of facts, it exposes the political and social processes through which they are constituted. Moreover, privileging 'matters of concern' over 'matters of fact' enables a richer account of phenomena as simultaneously socially constructed and thoroughly material. This book has been an attempt to reread (and hence remake) HIV as a matter of concern. It has theorised HIV as always already produced in discourse, yet no less real or agentive for being thus produced. Understood as a material-discursive phenomenon, HIV is constituted in practice; it is thus both an effect of social and political forces and helps to produce these forces. So instead of focusing on what discourse (including politics) does to matter or vice versa, the analysis proceeded on the premise that discourse and matter are co-constituted. Doing so discloses a radically different ontology of the disease HIV than would an objectivist realist approach. It reveals the materiality of HIV as politically constituted, that is, as emergent, rather than foundational. Here we might turn once more to Barad's (2007) concept of 'intra-action' to pose HIV as made and changed in its *intra-actions* with other material-discursive phenomena (themselves multiply co-constituted and open to change).

If one accepts that different intra-actions will materialise HIV differently, then it follows that disease, like all phenomena, is ontologically multiple. In this sense, and following Mol (2002, p. 5), we can understand disease as 'more than one and less than many', enacted multiply in daily practices across various sites but somehow managing to cohere as an apparently unified object. Crucially, the multiplicity and open-endedness of disease means that disease and its effects can be made differently. When one considers that stigma, political conflict and preventable suffering have accompanied HIV in South Africa, the possibility of making HIV differently should hold some appeal. Before offering some suggestions (however tentative and modest) for how HIV might be remade in ways that are responsible, generous and compassionate to those living with the disease, I draw together the main threads of the argument developed in the preceding chapters about the ontology of HIV and those living with it. My aim in doing so is to revisit the central theoretical concerns of the book, comment on the open-ended future of HIV/AIDS in South Africa and, finally, make some recommendations for how we (along with other 'non-human' participants) might help to shape this future. Importantly though, and breaking with convention, this closing chapter does not seek to offer a neat, comprehensive account spelling out the definitive conclusions that can be drawn from an analysis of the politics of HIV in South Africa. Neither does it make any claims to completeness or to simple answers, except perhaps to acknowledge that insofar as HIV is a site of contestation and struggle, its ontology is always already political. Eschewing the seductiveness of a tidy close, I make an effort here to remain faithful to the complexities and multiplicity of HIV. To do so is, I think, important because it preserves the tensions articulated in the debate and, indeed in the undulating course of HIV in South Africa.

Making disease and its subjects

At its heart, the theoretical approach taken in this book has been directed towards querying some of the enduring assumptions about the politics of HIV in South Africa and the fiercely contested debate over HIV that took place under former president Mbeki. In a departure from the existing scholarship on the South African HIV debate, the book has hinged on the central premise that the politics of the debate cannot be readily dismissed as irrelevant to the ontology of HIV in South Africa. Rather, the debate and the activity (and inactivity) it generated has materially shaped the disease and those living with it in specific and often damaging ways. In making this argument, four main lines of inquiry, corresponding with the key questions animating this book have been pursued in the preceding discussion. These are:

1. the ways in which politics makes the disease HIV;
2. the role of South Africa's colonial-apartheid history in producing specific, sometimes damaging, materialisations of HIV;
3. how the problem of HIV has been understood and the effects of particular problematisations on the relational field of HIV in South Africa;
4. the role of politics (including the HIV debate) in constituting subjects.

In terms of the first line of inquiry, this book is nothing less than an attempt to imagine and therefore help to constitute HIV differently. Over time, and through specific practices and the complex workings of politics, HIV is subject to change and this book is one small contribution to this process of change. It has sought to denaturalise but not entirely erase the taken-for-granted polarisation of the TAC–government debate over HIV, arguing that it is possible to see important continuities, rather than only differences, in the Mbeki government's and TAC's accounts of the disease. As I have demonstrated, the most significant continuity observed in their positions (and perhaps the one that shores up the others), is their understanding of HIV as a 'matter of fact' – a pre-formed object possessed of intrinsic characteristics that the 'right' kind of science can reveal. By reiterating the dualisms of nature/culture and biology/society, TAC and the government enacted HIV as either the product of nature, as in TAC's conceptualisation, or the product of culture, as in the government's formulation. Yet both accounts prove inadequate in the face of the disease's complexity: AIDS cannot be understood only as a syndrome caused by a virus (a biological or naturally given object), nor merely as a symptom of social factors like poverty and racial differences, which appear difficult to change. By holding fast to these foundational dualisms, these accounts preclude, or at least limit, the possibility of understanding HIV/AIDS as always already an assemblage of biological and social, natural and cultural forces. Furthermore, both accounts – in their intra-actions with each other and with the presumption of a polarised debate – actually did little to combat HIV as they held South Africa in aspic as it were, paralysing the national response and impeding action on the epidemic.

Furthermore, speaking of the facts of HIV as though they are self-evident and immutable obscures the constructedness and instability of facts. One could say then that the debate *reduces* HIV to a matter of fact, consistently eliding evidence of its contingency, dynamism and open-endedness. Perhaps most importantly, by posing disease as a pre-existing entity, the debate brackets out how practices (including those associated with the debate itself) help to materially constitute HIV as disease. As we have seen, the debate and the kinds of activity/inactivity it produces have shaped the substance of HIV and thus the epidemic in South Africa. For instance, the framing of the discussion in terms of the medical/social dualism tended to pushed policy prescriptions towards one side of the dualism, neglecting the other. This tendency is perhaps most clearly evident in the Mbeki government's emphasis on social-behavioural responses, at the expense of medical ones (notably, ART). Against the debate's rendering of disease as a matter of fact, the analysis conducted in the preceding chapters has sought to query the self-evidency of the 'facts of HIV' and reveal the role of politics in making disease and its facts. In doing so, it has not simply traced the various moves in the HIV debate in an effort to adjudicate on which facts about the disease are correct and will reveal some underlying 'truth' of HIV. Instead, it has been concerned to track just some of the many political phenomena that gathered together to produce specific material enactments of HIV/AIDS in South Africa during Mbeki's presidency (1999–2008) and in the years after it (2009–12).

In Chapter 2, I suggested that an agential realist approach generates new questions, beyond the conventional ones that assume HIV is a stable, fixed object, part of an unmediated nature. The recognition that disease is an emergent, multiply co-constituted phenomenon served as the conceptual lynchpin for the book's second line of inquiry: a careful tracking of how HIV has materialised in ways specific to post-apartheid South Africa. As each of the preceding chapters shows us, these materialisations emerge in relation to (and are thus ontologically inseparable from) the current and past politics of South Africa. Some of the key phenomena that constitute this politics include:

- the twin legacies of apartheid and colonialism;
- the racially discriminatory public health policies of the colonial and apartheid governments;
- the denigration of African sexuality in some Western scientific discourses;
- Mbeki's AIDS dissidence;
- the apparent polarisation of state–civil society responses to HIV under Mbeki;
- widespread poverty in South Africa;
- a reliance on a Western liberal conception of the 'human'; and
- the concurrence of the epidemic in South Africa with the transition from apartheid.

In tracking the role of these phenomena in producing specific enactments of HIV, I am not suggesting that they merely *inter*act with HIV to make the epidemic more severe or difficult to treat in South Africa but rather that these phenomena *intra*-actively constitute HIV and are themselves constituted by it. The point here is that these so-called external, political phenomena are inextricably entangled with the ontologies of the disease in South Africa. The analysis conducted in the preceding chapters is a reminder that there is a complex political history embedded in HIV in South Africa and if the disease is to be radically reconstituted, it is critical that we keep in focus the role of politics in differentially making HIV and its subjects.

The book's third line of inquiry centres on how the 'problem of HIV/AIDS' was variously formulated in the debate. As outlined in Chapter 2, Mbeki drew a series of connections between the problem of HIV/AIDS in South Africa and what he metaphorically termed the 'disease of racism', a metaphor that has historical underpinnings in apartheid's racially discriminatory public health policies. In an effort to elaborate on the contention that ideas about disease (here, a metaphor) partake in *making* the realities of disease, I argued that, by figuring racism as a disease, Mbeki rendered equivalent the struggle against one disease (HIV) with the struggle against another (racism). In the process he constituted racism as a lethal threat to South Africa's nascent democracy, deserving of equal or greater public consideration than the problem of the HIV epidemic. By prioritising the problem of racism and minimising that of HIV, Mbeki deflected attention and resources away from the HIV epidemic, allowing HIV infection and mortality rates to increase, thus helping to produce a materially altered epidemic, one that was more severe than it might otherwise have been.

Building on the analysis of problem representations presented in Chapter 2, Chapter 3 addressed the Mbeki government's problematisation of AIDS as a disease of poverty. Several problem representations are nested within this account. By posing AIDS as a socioeconomic problem (rather than a medical one), the government connected it with Africa's legacy of colonialism and its political economy of underdevelopment. These nested accounts of the problem of AIDS enact disease as the product of socio-political forces, an enactment that the TAC, at times, contested in positing disease as primarily the product of biological forces. TAC leaders argued that, although poverty contributes to AIDS, it is most properly seen as an infection with a clear biological cause in the form of a virus. Despite these differences, an important similarity exists in TAC's and the government's accounts of HIV: they both rely on the biological/social dualism, disease as either biological or social in origin. Because the debate was presented as bifurcated along orthodox/dissident lines, biological and social accounts of disease tended to be seen not only as distinct, but also as incompatible. Indeed, the key actors in the debate held fast to the bifurcation, making it difficult for either to concede any common ground in their positions. Yet it is possible to avoid reiterating the presumed ontological distinction between the biological and the social and to understand disease as a thoroughly biosocial phenomenon. At stake in this refiguring is the very substance of disease and the effectiveness of the measures taken to address it. As long as disease is understood via binary categories, such as biological/social and natural/cultural, it will continue to be taken as a natural (or biologically given) phenomenon, which precedes society, politics and culture. The performative role of social, political and cultural forces in *making* disease will thus remain unexamined, limiting the effectiveness of the measures taken to address it.

Lastly, in turning to the matter of how the subjects of HIV are differentially produced, the book has theorised HIV as a phenomenon iteratively made in practice, which enacts and is enacted by subjects. HIV-positive subjects are variously interpellated (and thus constituted) in the South African debate as victims of HIV, victims of poverty, vectors of disease, at-risk populations and agentive health citizens. The subject is thus revealed as dynamic and contingent, like disease itself. This is an important point because it means that there is nothing inevitable about the concentration of HIV among particular populations in South Africa, such as the rural poor, sex workers, young black women and migrant workers. Rather, the formation of particular kinds of subjects and patterns of vulnerability to HIV is, at least in part, an effect of specific (sometimes damaging) ideas about disease, policy decisions, scientific practices and public health measures. I am taken by the implicit recognition here that disease and its subjects could always be otherwise because in it lies the promise of generating different, less stigmatising versions of HIV and, with them, new selves for those affected by the disease. This book has been concerned to chart some of the existing enactments of HIV and those living with it in South Africa. Of course, and as I have ventured at various points in the preceding discussion, the exercise of producing what Rose (2007, p. 5) calls a 'cartography of [... the] present' is inspired by a belief that doing so might enable a different, more generous future. The final section of this conclusion offers some reflections on the agential possibilities for forging such a future of HIV in South Africa.

In pursuing these four key lines of inquiry, I have also sought to challenge the self-evidence of key phenomena bound up with the politics of HIV, such as the human, the citizen and the notions of responsibility and agency. Chapters 3 and 4, for example, addressed a series of questions about TAC's promotion of biological citizenship:

- What is a biological citizen and on what basis are attributions of citizenship made?
- On what logic does biological citizenship rely and how does this logic differentially constitute those living with HIV?
- What material effects might accompany the denial of citizenship?
- How does biological citizenship relate to the politics of life and death?

Across the two chapters, I developed the argument that the individualising and responsibilising norms of biological citizenship would seem to disqualify socially and materially marginalised HIV-positive subjects from full citizenship and therefore from being considered fully human. These marginalised others could all too easily become the casualties of biological citizenship, left to die by virtue of their perceived failure to consistently meet the requirements of citizenship. They also help to shape HIV/AIDS, producing at least two quite different – but co-constituted – enactments of the disease: a chronic, manageable disease for those who achieve citizen status, and an acute, fatal one for those who cannot consistently enact the attributes of the model citizen and who therefore cannot access the rights and rewards attendant on citizenship status.

Given the exclusions that can emerge through technologies of biological citizenship, it is important to interrogate its normative ideals of individual responsibility and unfettered agency in terms of their potential to disqualify certain subjects from full citizenship and thus from claiming the right to health care. Challenging the view that treats agency as an attribute of individual human subjects, I have proposed instead an extended conception of agency, one which sees it as a phenomenon produced in the encounters of humans and non-humans. Such a conception recognises that the human subject is not exclusively responsible for whether and how they conform to the norms of health citizenship. Seeing responsibility as distributed allows a more generous, nuanced understanding of HIV and its subjects. For example, it enables an account of treatment adherence framed not in terms of moralising judgements of patient fallibility, but rather in terms of the multiplicity of human and non-human forces that enable or constrain adherence. These forces include the design of treatment itself, reliable access to drugs, the attitudes of health practitioners, the operation of medical supply chains and the management of the public health system. Instead of trying to make HIV-positive patients 'more responsible', there remains cause to consider how the ethics of biomedicine might change if responsibility were understood as distributed across the human and non-human continuum. This extended notion of responsibility is not confined to the issue of biological citizenship. It has broader significance and pertains to the HIV debate too. Seeing responsibility as distributed enables a rethinking of the positions articulated in debate, disrupting their assumed polarisation and seeing them instead not only as mutually constituted but also mutually responsible for helping to make HIV and those living with it in South Africa.

One of the book's abiding concerns has been to subject to careful scrutiny the Cartesian dualisms implicit in the debate (nature/culture, matter/meaning, human/non-human and so on). The analysis conducted in Chapter 4 examined the human/non-human dualism, asking the deceptively simple question, what is a human? How is the human defined against the spectre of the non-human? Given that the legal battle for public sector ART in South Africa was fought on the grounds of human rights, and appeals to rights continue to be taken as self-evidently just and thus considered above criticism, it seems a pressing scholarly task to disturb received notions of the human and question whether the ideal of human rights is as fair and inclusive as liberal Enlightenment politics would have us believe. Who is the privileged subject of human rights? What exclusions accompany rights claims? In addressing this issue, I elaborated on the connections between TAC's rights-based struggle for HIV treatment and its promotion of biological citizenship, observing the co-constitution of the human and the (biological) citizen and their presumed binary opposites, the non-human and the non-citizen. As we have seen these binaries reciprocally constitute each other to produce certain HIV-positive subjects as (fully human) biological citizens and to disqualify others from citizenship, thereby excluding them from the domain of the fully human.

Remaking HIV in South Africa: some agential possibilities

If the destructive course of HIV in South Africa is to be radically altered, there is value in pursuing strategies attuned to the performative work of politics (including the strategies themselves) in making and changing the disease. At various points in the book, I have gestured towards some of the measures that might facilitate such change. Here I wish to consolidate the kinds of actions I have suggested would help to make HIV differently. In remaking the disease, I, like others, envisage doing so in ways that help prevent new infections and that thwart the development of drug-resistant strains of the virus. Whenever the disease is remade, its treatment is too. So, in imagining that the relational field of HIV might be otherwise, the book calls for enactments of HIV treatment that challenge the status of ART as an 'unsatisfactory privilege' (Rosengarten, 2009, p. 103), in the sense that it is still not available to most of those in need and, where it is available, it demands stringent adherence and can induce debilitating side-effects. In short, I envisage remaking HIV as part of a politics of life, one which is governed by the impulse to 'make live', and which guards against its corresponding latent capacity to 'let die' (Foucault, 2003, p. 241).

The politics of life proposed here, resonates with, but also departs from, Rose's critical take on what he calls the 'politics of life itself' (2007, p. 40). Rose's approach concerns the role of contemporary biopolitics in producing human beings as 'somatic individuals' (Rose, 2007, p. 26), whose bodies and lives are open to choice, experimentation, and continual management and optimisation. Although we are both interested in the political practices and processes by which subjects are made to live (or consigned to death), Rose appears to take the human as a self-evident starting point for his analysis. The politics of life envisaged here might productively employ Barad's post-humanist performativity – perhaps along with other post-humanist approaches – to challenge the self-evidence of the human and to explore the differential constitution of humans and non-humans. Crucially, as a post-humanist formulation, this politics would be responsive to the role of human and non-human forces in materialising HIV and those living with the disease. Consistent with Barad's (2007) post-humanist ethics, it would see agency, not as an attribute of individual human subjects but as distributed across humans and non-humans. Such a rethinking of agency enables an account that avoids locating culpability or failure unjustly and simplistically in the actions (or inaction) of individual human subjects. For example, instead of attributing poor treatment outcomes to individual subjects' failure to adhere to stringent drug regimes, we would do better to attend to the diverse array of co-constituted forces (or as Barad would put it, 'intra-actions') through which treatment success/failure is produced.

Remaking HIV as part of a politics of life has important implications for the design of public health policy and practice. It would require policy to be critically reflexive, that is, always alert and responsive to its role in producing specific, sometimes damaging enactments of HIV and affected individuals. Somewhat paradoxically, disease concepts and policies developed as part of a politics of life would be attentive, not only to the numbers of lives saved, but also to those needlessly lost to HIV in an era when life-prolonging treatment is available, if still only to some of those in need. The formulation of ethical responses to disease necessitates asking the uncomfortable question: how are particular ideas about disease implicated in producing certain lives as less worthy/unworthy? In short, how do our theories (and hence practices) partake in allowing certain subjects to live with HIV, consigning others to die from AIDS?

Lest the vision articulated above appear merely a utopian fantasy, I make some suggestions for the kinds of conceptual shifts and actions that would be helpful in remaking HIV within a politics of life. To begin with, and following policy theorist Carol Bacchi (2009), it is helpful to consider the question: how could we understand (and therefore produce) the problem differently and why might it be helpful to do so? As we have seen, the HIV debate framed the policy problem in terms of the 'facts' of HIV and how best to 'respond' to the disease on the basis of these apparent facts. This view of the problem presumes that disease precedes human action and that humans merely intervene to ameliorate its effects. Against this conventional view, I suggest framing the problem in terms of the broader relational field within which a disease like HIV is produced and changed. Doing so invites the recognition that the 'facts' of HIV are temporary and contingent, produced in relation to (rather than preceding) human action. This reframing of the problem also entails acknowledging the generative work of *non-human* participants in making disease. In this respect, it follows Barad's (2007) post-humanist performativity, which addresses the role of both humans and non-humans (hence 'post-humanist') in the making of realities (hence 'performativity'). For example, and as we saw in Chapters 2, 3 and 4, putatively non-human phenomena such as drugs, condoms, the availability of flush toilets, viral load counts and an overburdened public health system play a crucial role in materialising HIV in South Africa. With this in mind, it is necessary to engage the performative work of specific human and non-human phenomena in producing harmful enactments of the disease. Only then can we consider how we might remake the disease, alleviate its effects and, in so doing, remake the multiple phenomena with which it is entangled. These include, but are certainly not limited to: poverty, citizenship, the human, treatment, prevention, epidemiology, public health, science, ethics, global inequalities, race, the HIV-positive subject, sexual practices and stigma. When the disease changes, these phenomena – and doubtless many others not listed here – do too. Therefore much can be gained by refiguring HIV in terms that move beyond the apparently immutable facts of the disease and that engage instead the politics (or broader relational field) within which the disease is continually made and changed.

Had the TAC and the government taken this view of disease, it might have allowed the HIV debate to be conducted differently, without being framed in terms of traditional dualisms, such as nature/culture, biological/social, human/non-human and so on. Importantly, as the preceding chapters have shown, the assumption of a polarised debate did little to resolve the problem of HIV as it effectively froze the national response, impeding the delivery of treatment until such time as those involved could agree on whose version of the 'truth' of HIV would prevail. Had the major actors in the debate recognised the ways in which statements of 'truth' are themselves part of the politics that makes HIV, it would have freed them to transcend the seemingly polarised debate about the 'facts' or 'truth' of HIV. Doing so might have allowed the TAC to concede the role of poverty and racist colonialism in shaping HIV/AIDS in South Africa. Furthermore, it might have enabled the government to acknowledge the importance of an imperfect medicine in treating the disease. In short, I suggest that had the debate been conducted following a more nuanced view of disease as a matter of concern – as always in the making, contingent on political, social and historical forces – it might have allowed both TAC and the government to avoid some of the persistent pitfalls and epistemic traps associated with treating disease as a simple matter of fact.

Given that HIV is a social-cultural phenomenon as much as a so-called natural one; responses to HIV need to jointly address the 'natural' and 'cultural' forces entangled with the disease and which help to produce it. In South Africa, this means engaging the ways in which poverty is often embodied in the ontologies of HIV and those living with the disease. It might involve, for example, the design of a treatment policy that works not only to ensure the successful delivery of ART, but also to redress the persistent social inequalities that shape the distribution and effects of HIV in South Africa. Such a policy holds considerable potential to promote better treatment adherence as it would operate on the assumption that responsibility for adherence is not the sole prerogative of individual human subjects but rather is distributed across human and non-human forces. As such, it could include provisions for the following, some of which are already being pursued by the

South African government and local civil society organisations, such as the TAC:

- universal basic income support (not limited to narrow definitions of unemployment, disability or viral load);
- formal housing;
- free public health care for all residents of South Africa (not only citizens);
- research on improved drug design;
- vaginal and anal microbicides as alternatives to male condoms (currently the main HIV prevention technology);
- monitoring and addressing mismanagement in the public health system; and
- promoting an even distribution of ART across all provincial health care sites.

Of course, the measures proposed here would require a substantial investment of state resources and raise the question of affordability. It is therefore important to reiterate that pursuing even just one or two of them would change other policy areas too. If we understand objects as multiply co-constituted phenomena, whatever investments are made on a particular phenomenon (here HIV) will extend to others. It is this insight that separates the measures I am suggesting from those that others, working within a conventional realist approach, have suggested.

The account of disease elaborated in this book prompts the recognition that, as with the phenomenon of poverty, HIV both embodies and (re)produces racial and gender inequalities in South Africa. Or, as Barad might put it, HIV, race and gender are made and changed in their intra-actions. In Chapter 2, I argued that HIV intra-acts with violent masculinities, massive youth unemployment, poverty and the vestiges of racial oppression to help produce an epidemic that disproportionately affects young black women in South Africa (Abdool Karim and Frolich, 2000). Conceiving the phenomena of race and gender as separate or irrelevant to the materiality of HIV is to neglect the ways in which they co-constitute the disease. The effectiveness of measures taken to address HIV can only be impeded by such a simplistic conception. Conversely, and as already noted, measures that address the co-constitution of HIV and related social-political phenomena (such as race and gender) will be more far-reaching than anticipated. The ameliorative effects will extend to other mutually constituted social problems, such as violent masculinities, poverty, the uneven disease burden on young black women, youth unemployment and high rates of violence against women. The kinds of measures that could enable these far-reaching effects include a more broadly defined affirmative action policy, one that is not restricted (as the current one is) to post-apartheid employment equity measures. Such a policy has the potential to redress disparities in health care along the lines of gender, race, socioeconomic status and nationality. It could work to ensure that all those living with HIV in South Africa – whether male or female, black or white, rich or poor, citizens or foreign residents – have equal and fair access to HIV prevention, screening and treatment. Adopting an affirmative action approach to health care might enable a fairer distribution of health care, and thus a more even HIV burden, across race, socioeconomic status, gender and nationality.

When disease is remade, its subjects are too. Therefore, in helping to produce more compassionate, generous enactments of HIV, we need to acknowledge that those living with the disease, and all of us who are in some way entangled with it, will be remade too. Importantly, because intra-actions do not operate on a linear causal logic, we cannot predict the ways in which we will be changed by our efforts to remake HIV. Following Race (2012, p. 336), I venture that we need, therefore, to learn to live with ontological indeterminacy, to 'giv[e] [.... ourselves] over to a shared but indeterminate future'. In short, and to return to a concept elaborated by Mol (1999, p. 74), I am calling for approaches to disease that engage, not only in a politics of life, but more broadly in 'ontological politics'. This book is one example of an ontological politics of disease: in rethinking HIV and challenging the self-evidence of influential ideas about the epidemic in South Africa, it makes a contribution, however small and incremental, to making the disease differently.

Disease, as we have seen, is not the simple product of nature or culture, science or politics. Neither is it reducible to the status of a non-human object which is presumed to infect an otherwise pure human subject. Disease can more usefully be understood as an assemblage of natural, cultural, human, non-human, scientific and political forces. Furthermore, insofar as disease is embodied in and inseparable from its (human) host, it is at once self and other, subject and object. Crucially, this book has emphasised the contingency of existing enactments of disease and the openness of future ones. It is this openness that allows me to finish on an optimistic note by returning to Barad's post-humanist ethics and citing her rousing appeal to participate in an ontological politics:

> The world and its possibilities for becoming are remade with each moment [...] Meeting each moment, being alive to the possibilities

of becoming is an ethical call, an invitation that is written into the very matter of all being and becoming. (Barad, 2008, p. 396)

The search for new ways of addressing HIV can only be strengthened by the recognition that the ontology of the disease is contingent, open-ended and multiple. We, along with other differentially constituted human and non-human participants, can help to forge different, kinder enactments of HIV, if only we accept the risk that we too will be altered in unanticipated ways by our efforts.

Appendix A: An Overview of the Struggles over HIV in South Africa (1998–2014)

10 December 1998 – The Treatment Action Campaign (TAC), led by South African HIV activist Zackie Achmat, announces its formation and stages a protest with the National Association of People with AIDS (NAPWA) for a 'comprehensive and affordable treatment plan for all people living with HIV/AIDS' (Geffen, 2010, p. 49).

June 1999 – Thabo Mbeki is elected President of South Africa and Dr Mantombazana Tshabalala-Msimang is appointed Minister of Health.

28 October 1999 – Mbeki addresses Parliament on the HIV epidemic. He claims that anti-retroviral drugs (ARVs), in particular AZT, are toxic and 'a danger to health' (Heywood, 2005).

April 2000 – Mbeki writes a letter to leaders of the Group of Eight (G8) nations addressing the issue of HIV/AIDS. He calls for an African response to the epidemic, arguing that 'a simple superimposition of Western experience on African reality [...] would be absurd and illogical [...] a criminal betrayal of our responsibility to our own people' (Mbeki, 2000c).

May 2000 – President of the South African Medical Research Council, Professor Malegapuru Makgoba writes an editorial piece for the journal *Science* in which he criticises Mbeki's stance on HIV, denouncing it as absurd and pseudo-scientific. He calls for a logical, rational response to the South African HIV epidemic, 'lest history judges us to have collaborated in one of the greatest crimes of our time' (Makgoba, 2000, para. 6).

6–7 May 2000 (Durban) and 3–4 July 2000 (Johannesburg) – Mbeki convenes the 'Presidential Advisory Panel on AIDS' to review the science on HIV/AIDS (Youdé, 2007a). The panel comprises international and local scientists. Two-thirds of the panel are proponents of mainstream HIV/AIDS science and the remaining panellists are AIDS dissidents (Youdé, 2007a). Ten members of the AIDS dissident group issue a 'Minority Statement', making the following assertions:

1. AIDS is not contagious, although many of the opportunistic manifestations are;
2. AIDS is not sexually transmitted;
3. AIDS is not caused by HIV;
4. the admittedly toxic anti-HIV drugs are killing people;
5. the drug-induced toxic effects are causing AIDS-defining conditions that cannot be distinguished from AIDS. (Bialy *et al.*, 2000, paras 1–5)

July 2000 – In the run-up to the Thirteenth International AIDS Conference and in response to the public disputes of the Presidential Advisory Panel, physicians and scientists from 82 countries sign the 'Durban Declaration' affirming the validity of scientific research on AIDS and stating that the findings are 'compelling' and 'exhaustive' (Durban Declaration: A Declaration by Scientists and Physicians Affirming HIV is the Cause of AIDS, 2000, pp. 15–16). In his opening address at the conference, Mbeki states:

> The world's biggest killer and the greatest cause of ill health and suffering across the globe, including South Africa, is extreme poverty [...] As I listened and heard the whole story about our own country, it seemed to me that we could not blame everything on a single virus. (Mbeki, 2000d)

21 August 2000 – A 25-year-old HIV-positive woman, Mpho Motloung is murdered by her husband in Soweto, a township south-west of Johannesburg. A note is left on her body that reads, 'HIV Positive AIDS'. In an official statement, TAC chairperson Zackie Achmat links Mpho's murder to the discrimination, fear and confusion surrounding HIV/AIDS in South Africa, arguing that this climate of fear and stigma promotes violence against openly HIV-positive people (Achmat, 2000).

11 September 2000 – In an interview with *Time Magazine*, Mbeki is questioned on his views on the causal link between HIV and AIDS. He replies, stating:

> If you go through the literature, ordinary standard literature available in medical schools, there will be a whole variety of things that can cause the immune system to collapse. Endemic poverty, the impact of

nutrition, contaminated water, all those things will result in immune deficiency. If you take the African context, you add things like repetitive infections of malaria, syphilis, gonorrhea etc. All of these things will result in immune deficiency. Now, it is perfectly possible that among those things is a particular virus. (Mbeki, 2000, cited in Fassin, 2007, p. 31)

17 September 2000 – The government issues a statement emphasising that the President and his Cabinet do not deny the link between HIV and AIDS. The full transcript of the *Time Magazine* interview is posted on the African National Congress (ANC) website, along with a statement claiming that the President had been quoted out of context: 'The context of the full transcript makes it expressly clear that he was prepared to accept that HIV might "very well" be a casual factor' (Government statement, 2000, cited in Fassin, 2007, p. 31).

April 2001 – The South African Medicines Control Council (MCC) registers the ARV drug Nevirapine for use in the prevention of mother-to-child transmission (PMTCT) (Patterson, 2006). But the Department of Health expresses concerns about its safety and efficacy and decides to test the drug in a pilot study at two sites in each of the country's nine provinces. The study targets 18 hospitals, reaching an estimated 10 per cent of HIV-positive pregnant women in need of the drug (Patterson, 2006).

24 April 2001 – Mbeki announces on national TV that he will not be taking a public HIV test, stating: 'I go and do a test – I am confirming a particular paradigm' (Mbeki, 2001, cited in van der Vliet, 2004, p. 63).

August 2001 – The TAC initiates legal action against the government for failing to extend public access to PMTCT beyond the pilot sites, arguing that its failure to do so violates the right to health care (Hodes, 2011).

14 December 2001 – In the case of the *Treatment Action Campaign and Others v Minister of Health and Others* on the matter of PMTCT, the South African High Court rules that the government has an obligation to deliver a national PMTCT programme: 'About one thing there must be no misunderstanding: a countrywide MTCT prevention program is an ineluctable obligation of the state' (Botha, 2001, cited in van der Vliet, 2004, p. 70).

January 2001 – The Minister of Health appeals the High Court judgment, arguing that the court does not have the jurisdiction to decide on health policy. The matter is referred to the Constitutional Court.

February 2002 – The tide of opinion within the government begins to shift as former political allies of the Mbeki administration register their discontent with the national HIV policy. Minister of Home Affairs and leader of the opposition Inkatha Freedom Party (IFP) Mangosuthu Buthelezi express concerns over the government's decision not to deliver a national PMTCT programme.

5 July 2002 – The Constitutional Court rules in support of the High Court judgment and orders the government to develop and implement a comprehensive PMTCT programme.

December 2002 – Provision of PMTCT remains patchy across South Africa and the TAC launches a contempt of court application against Mpumulanga Member of the Executive Council, Dr Sibongile Manana for not implementing the court order in her province (Heywood, 2003). The application implicates national Health Minister Tshabalala-Msimang for failing to ensure all provinces complied with the court order.

March 2003 – The TAC launches a civil disobedience campaign to pressure the government to deliver a national ART programme (Low et al., 2010). Titled 'Dying for Treatment', the campaign includes protests, marches, pickets and laying a charge of culpable homicide against the Minister of Health for not implementing ART in the public health sector.

July 2003 – HIV-positive TAC leader, Zackie Achmat protests against the government's refusal to deliver a national ART programme, announcing that he will not be taking ART until it is available to all South Africans (Low et al., 2010).

August 2003 – The government accedes to the pressure from TAC and other civil society organisations to deliver ART and begins to roll out ART in public hospitals (Low et al., 2010).

November 2003 – The South African Cabinet approves the country's first Comprehensive HIV/AIDS Care Management and Treatment Plan. The plan commits to the delivery of a nationwide ART programme.

13 December 2003 – 22-year-old TAC member and treatment literacy educator, Lorna Mlofana is gang raped and murdered after revealing her HIV status (Low et al., 2010).

April 2004 – After the second democratic election, when the ANC is re-elected ruling party, President Mbeki announces his government's commitment to ensuring that ART reaches 53,000 people with HIV.

June 2004 – The TAC estimates suggest that fewer than 10,000 South Africans are on state-funded HIV treatment.

August 2006 – The South African stand at the International AIDS Conference in Toronto provokes outrage from delegates and HIV activists. Health Minister Tshabalala-Msimang is responsible for the exhibition stall, which promotes beetroot, garlic and other remedies as alternative treatments for HIV (Jones, 2009). In the closing address of the AIDS conference, the chairperson Dr Mark Wainberg chastises Health Minister Tshabalala-Msimang for South Africa's HIV policy and calls for her immediate dismissal:

> To have as Health Minister a person who now has no international respect is an embarrassment to the South African government. We therefore call for the immediate removal of Dr Tshabalala-Msimang as Minister of Health, and for an end to the disastrous, pseudo-scientific policies that have characterised the South African government's response to HIV/AIDS. (Wainberg 2006, cited in Afrolnews, 2006)

October 2006 – According to national statistics, 224,895 HIV-positive South Africans are on ART.

April 2007 – The Ministry of Health implements a National Strategic Plan (NSP) to address HIV. Encompassing the period 2007 to 2011, it includes provisions for 'expanding access to appropriate treatment, care and support to 80 per cent of all HIV positive people and their families by 2011' (South African National Aids Council, 2007, p. 29). Between 2007 and 2011, South Africa increases its HIV treatment services by 75 per cent (Shisana *et al.*, 2014).

21 September 2008 – President Mbeki delivers his final 'Address to the Nation' before stepping down as President after the ANC called for him to resign because he attempted to prosecute Deputy President Jacob Zuma for corruption.

May 2009 – Jacob Zuma is elected as President of South Africa, signalling for many the end of state-supported AIDS dissidence in South Africa (TAC, 2009).

October 2009 – President Zuma delivers a speech in which he acknowledges HIV as a profound challenge confronting South Africa and calls for an urgent, concerted response to the epidemic: 'We need to move with urgency and purpose to confront this enormous challenge [...]

Most importantly, all South Africans need to know their HIV status, and be informed of the treatment options available to them' (Zuma, 2009).

2012 – A report commissioned by the Human Sciences Research Council (HSRC) based on national survey data estimates that 6.4 million South Africans or 12.6 per cent are living with HIV, an increase in prevalence from three previous surveys conducted between 2002 and 2008 (Shisana *et al.*, 2014). HSRC Chief Executive Officer Olive Shisana attributes the slightly increased prevalence rate to the four-fold increase in the number of people on HIV treatment who are surviving and thus 'swelling the number of people living with HIV' (Shisana, 2014, cited in Maurice, 2014, p. 1535).

2014 – Following the adoption of the second NSP on HIV (2011–13), which mandated the scale-up of ART, South Africa now has the biggest ART programme in the world and spends over $1 billion annually on its HIV programmes. Current Health Minister Aaron Motsolaedi describes South Africa's future HIV policy and practice as being directed towards a 'combination HIV prevention' programme:

> No one method alone can defeat this epidemic. My strategy for the future is to bring together in a coordinated manner all the different means we have of dealing with the epidemic – communicating, promoting condom use, getting more men to accept medical circumcision, developing a post-exposure prophylaxis programme, increasing the numbers of infected people on ART, and so on. Accelerating combination prevention is my priority now. (Motsolaedi, 2014, cited in Maurice, 2014, p. 1536)

Notes

Introduction: HIV/AIDS as a Site of Struggle in South Africa

1. According to the accepted biomedical definition, the Human Immunodeficiency Virus (HIV) is the virus that causes Acquired Immune Deficiency Syndrome (AIDS) (Centers for Disease Control and Prevention [CDC], 2006). HIV is transmitted through exchange of blood, genital fluids or breast milk. It can also be transmitted from mother to child during pregnancy or delivery. AIDS is a cluster of diseases and opportunistic infections that break down the body's immune defences, hence the term 'immunodeficiency'. AIDS-related illnesses and infections are thus symptomatic of a compromised immune system and may include tuberculosis, diarrhoea, pneumonia, Karposi's sarcoma and fungal infections. Following the medical distinction drawn between HIV and AIDS, I use 'AIDS' to refer to the late stage of HIV infection where the immune system is severely compromised, as indicated by a low white blood cell count and/or by the presence of AIDS-related opportunistic infections such as tuberculosis, diarrhoea and pneumonia. The term 'HIV' is used to denote the virus that helps to produce AIDS. In all other cases, I use the term 'HIV/AIDS' to refer jointly to the virus and the syndrome, that is, to the disease, more generally. This last usage is intended to capture the enduring association between HIV and AIDS in contexts where, for example, anti-retroviral treatment (ART) is not available and/or where poverty and other phenomena prevent a decoupling of the two.
2. ART or highly active anti-retroviral therapy (HAART) comprises a combination of three or more ARV drugs to treat HIV (WHO [World Health Organization], 2013). ARV drugs suppress the replication of HIV, allowing the immune system to recover. However, they do not entirely kill the virus and so ART is a long-term form of treatment. For the purposes of brevity, I refer to this form of treatment simply as ART or HIV treatment.
3. Mol (1999) credits John Law with coining the term 'ontological politics'. She then developed the concept in her paper entitled 'Ontological Politics: A Word and Some Questions'.
4. Consistent with the 'ontological' turn in contemporary social theory, new materialist approaches emphasise the agency of matter in the making of realities (Dolphijn and van der Tuin, 2012; Lezaun, 2014). They also conceive of the process of materialisation as ongoing, complex and contingent on social and political forces. On this view, social actors and theorists actively help to make realities and therefore the practices and concepts they employ have performative power: they bring certain realities into being and foreclose the existence of others.
5. For example, the work of Fraser and Seear (2011) and Seear (2014).

1 Disease in Theory and Practice

1. CD4 stands for Cluster of Differentiation Four and is a type of white blood cell (or T-cell) that assists with the body's immune response (WebMD, 2012). The number of CD4 cells per cubic millilitre (mm^3) of blood is seen as an indicator of the capacity of the immune system to manage infection. HIV is believed to bind to the surface of CD4 cells and then enters these cells, where it is able to replicate as the CD4 cells replicate. Gradually, as the virus replicates, the number of CD4 cells declines and the body's immune system response becomes compromised. A normal CD4 count is 500–1500 cells/mm^3. Counts below 200 are considered low and, in such cases, it is recommended that anti-retroviral therapy (ART) be started. The aim of ART is to suppress viral replication and maintain CD4 counts in the normal range of 500–1500/mm^3.
2. The idea of human identity contributing to its own infectious defeat could function as a metaphor for understanding Mbeki's response to HIV. Extending Waldby's metaphor, we might describe South Africa's colonial past as forcing it to embrace 'alien' ideas in the form of (Western) humanism, which meant the nation (as 'self') 'participated in its own infectious defeat' from HIV/AIDS (as 'other'). For a detailed discussion of Mbeki's appeals to Western humanism and the role of colonialism in shaping HIV in South Africa, see the analysis in Chapter 4.
3. As Waldby points out, immunology's depiction of 'self' and 'other' as binarily opposed is selective because 'under other representational conditions immunology acknowledges the importance of "benign" yet foreign micro-organisms that help in the regulation of the body's interior environment – in the gut, the mouth and so on' (Waldby, 1996, p. 64).

2 Contesting Science, Making Disease

1. In an ANC newsletter article reflecting on the issues raised in the parliamentary debate, Mbeki cursorily mentions the issue of rape, referring to it using the vague technical term, 'contact crime':

   > For those genuinely interested and involved in the national effort to improve the safety and security of our people, the crime statistics must indicate that more work needs to be done to prevent the commission of these 'contact crimes' especially in their areas of concentration, as identified by the Crime Statistics. (Mbeki, 2004a, para. 11)

   As with the case of the parliamentary debate, Mbeki's choice of language generalises rape; it fails to acknowledge that rape is an act of gender-based violence, distinguishing it from other 'contact crimes' such as physical assault and aggravated robbery.
2. So, according to Barad's model, 'race' and 'violent masculinities' are themselves the effect of intra-actions, just as HIV is.
3. For examples of this depiction, see Kalichman (2009), Makgoba (2002) and Geffen (2005).
4. Path-breaking feminist science studies research includes that of Haraway (1989), Harding (1986, 1991), Keller (1985) and Martin (1996).

5. Castro Hlongwane was a black South African boy who was the target of racial discrimination in a caravan park. He was ordered to leave by the park owner, who allegedly expressed concerns that Castro had HIV and would rape other residents of the park.
6. Feminist philosopher Sandra Harding (1991, p. 1) refers to positivist science as 'science as usual' in recognition of its hegemonic status.
7. Germ theory holds that micro-organisms (pathogens) are the underlying causal agents of most diseases.
8. In South Africa, the term 'coloured' refers to people of mixed race who are considered neither 'black' nor 'white' nor 'Indian', according to the apartheid racial categories. The apartheid system delineated 'coloured' as an apparently distinct racial group, classifying an ethnically diverse range of people according to this category by virtue of their mixed ancestry.
9. See for example, Mbali (2004), Wang (2004) and Fassin (2007).
10. Unlike the traditional Cartesian cuts that take binary oppositions as given, agential cuts enact or produce ontological boundaries (Barad, 2007).
11. Gieryn's (1995) notion of boundary-work resonates with Barad's (2007) agential realist account of the intra-active constitution of boundaries. Both scholars understand boundaries as performatively constituted, although it could be argued that Barad's account of boundaries as the effect of specific agential cuts is more sophisticated. The consistency in their approaches is suggested by the shared language of 'boundary-work': where Gieryn (1995, p. 405) refers to the 'boundary-work of science', Barad (2007, p. 140) refers to 'boundary-drawing practices', which she defines as 'specific material (re)configurings of the world'.

3 Poverty in the Making of HIV/AIDS

1. In this context, the 'omnipotent apparatus' refers to the international AIDS orthodoxy or what Youdé (2007a, p. 18) calls the 'international AIDS control regime', an epistemic community of Western scientists, public health practitioners, multinational pharmaceuticals, policy-makers, HIV/AIDS organisations and activists.
2. Some parts of Khayelitsha comprise formal housing and others (particularly the newer areas) comprise informal settlements with 70 per cent of residents living in corrugated metal and wooden shacks. It is estimated that one in three residents has to walk at least 200 metres to access clean water (Curry, 2011).
3. At 2015 exchange rates, 2000 South African Rand (ZAR) is equivalent to 104 British pounds (GBP) and 162 US dollars (USD). To put the cost of ARV drugs in perspective, a recent Quarterly Labour Force Survey estimated the average monthly earnings in South Africa to be R2800 (Statistics South Africa, 2010).
4. The TAC's emphasis on instating 'structure' in the life of a newly diagnosed HIV-positive person may also be a response to concerns expressed by some international leaders and policy-makers that ART regimens are 'too complex for Africans to adhere to'. The TAC and allied civil society organisations, such as Médecins Sans Frontières (MSF) sought to 'demonstrate that, with access to the correct information, antiretrovirals could be successfully rolled out in Africa' (Low et al., 2010, p. 35).

4 Disease as a Politics of the Human

1. See, for example, the work of early postcolonial scholars Frantz Fanon (1967a), Albert Memmi (1990) and Aimé Césaire (1955), which, despite their different emphases, all appeal to 'human solidarity' and to a racially inclusive understanding of the human.
2. Fanon's gender-blind language in his theorisation of a new humanism elides the gendered dynamics of traditional humanism, specifically its historical exclusion of women from the category human.
3. See Chapter 3 for more details of the case, including an analysis of the portrayal of HIV-positive pregnant women and their babies as innocent victims of the government's PMTCT policy. For an account of the background, legal arguments and outcomes of the case, see Heywood (2003).
4. The South African Department of Home Affairs estimates that there are between 2.5 million and 5 million undocumented migrants living in South Africa, although figures are unreliable (Crush and Williams, 2001). These migrants do not have temporary residence or asylum seeker permits, hence the term 'undocumented'. Although not entitled to access social services, undocumented migrants do have the right to emergency medical care, including ART (Crush and Williams, 2001). However, because they do not enjoy the rights and freedoms of citizens or documented migrants, they are very vulnerable and, as already noted, some evidence suggests they may be subject to 'medical xenophobia' when seeking medical care (Human Rights Watch, 2008).

Bibliography

Abdool Karim, S. and Abdool Karim, Q. (2005) *HIV/AIDS in South Africa*. Cambridge: Cambridge University Press.
Abdool Karim, Q. and Frolich, J. (2000) 'Women Try to Protect Themselves from HIV/AIDS in KwaZulu-Natal, South Africa', in Turshen, M. (ed.) *African Women's Health*. Lawrenceville, NJ: Africa World Press, pp. 243–261.
Achmat, Z. (2000) Treatment Action Campaign: Urgent Press Release (23 August 2000), at: www.tac.org.za/Documents/Statements/pr000823.txt (accessed 19 April 2013).
Afrolnews (2006) ' "Sack SA Health Minister" – World's AIDS Experts' (6 September 2006), at: www.afrol.com/articles/21094 (accessed 12 July 2015).
Amado, L. A., Christofides, N., Pieters, R. and Rusch, J. (2012) 'National Health Insurance: A Lofty Ideal in Need of Cautious, Planned Implementation', *South African Journal of Bioethics and Law* 5(1): 4–10.
Amon, J. and Todrys, K. (2009) 'Access to Antiretroviral Treatment for Migrant Populations in the Global South', *Sur – International Journal on Human Rights* 4: 154–177.
Anderson, K. (2007) *Race and the Crisis of Humanism*. Oxford: Routledge.
Angelides, S. (2011) 'Disorder as "Pseudo-Idea" ', *Atlantis: Critical Studies in Gender, Culture and Social Justice* 35(2): 10–20.
Annan, K. (2002) 'In Africa, AIDS Has a Woman's Face', *New York Times: International Herald Tribune*, at: www.un.org/News/ossg/sg/stories/sg-29dec-2002.htm (accessed 14 December 2011).
Anonymous (2002) 'Castro Hlongwane, Caravans, Cats, Geese, Foot and Mouth and Statistics: HIV/AIDS and the Struggle for the Humanisation of the African', at: www.virusmyth.com/aids/hiv/ancdoc.htm (accessed 12 August 2010).
AVERT (2008) *Worldwide HIV and AIDS statistics*, at: www.avert.org/worldstats.htm (accessed 11 August 2010).
AVERT (2011) *History of AIDS Up to 1986*, at: www.avert.org/aids-history-86.htm (accessed 3 November 2011).
Bacchi, C. L. (2009) *Analysing Policy: What's the Problem Represented to Be?* Frenchs Forest, NSW: Pearson.
Barad, K. (2003) 'Posthumanist Performativity: Toward an Understanding of How Matter Comes to Matter', *Signs* 28(3): 801–831.
Barad, K. (2007) *Meeting the Universe Halfway: Quantum Physics and the Entanglement of Matter and Meaning*. Durham, NC: Duke University Press.
Barad, K. (2008) 'Meeting the Universe Halfway: Feminism, Science and the Philosophy of Science', in Alaimo, S. and Hekman, S. (eds) *Material Feminisms*. Bloomington/Indianapolis: Bloomington University Press, pp. 120–154.
Bateman, C. (2013) 'Drug Stock-outs: Inept Supply-chain Management and Corruption', *SAMJ: South African Medical Journal* 103: 600–602.
Bauman, Z. (2003) 'The Project of Humanity', in Sheehan, P. (ed.) *Becoming Human: New Perspectives on the Inhuman Condition*. Westport, CT: Praeger, pp. 127–147.

Bayer, R. (1997) 'Review of *Impure Science: AIDS, Activism and the Politics of Knowledge*, by S. Epstein', *Science* 275(5298): 320.
Bialy, H., de Harven, E., Duesberg, P., Fiala, C., Giraldo, R., Herxheimer A. et al. (2000) 'Minority Statement and Recommendations to the Government of South Africa', at: www.virusmyth.com/aids/news/minorstat.htm (accessed 19 April 2013).
Biehl, J. G. (2004) 'The Activist State: Global Pharmaceuticals, AIDS, and Citizenship in Brazil', *Social Text* 22(3): 105–132.
Biehl, J. G. (2007) *Will to Live: AIDS Therapies and the Politics of Survival*. Princeton, NJ: Princeton University Press.
Boonzaier, F. (2005) 'Woman Abuse in South Africa: A Brief Contextual Analysis', *Feminism & Psychology* 15(1): 99–103.
Botha, J. (2001) *Treatment Action Campaign and Others v Minister of Health and Others*. Johannesburg: High Court of South Africa.
Butchart, A. (1998) *The Anatomy of Power: European Constructions of the African Body*. London: Zed Books.
Butler, A. (2005) 'South Africa's HIV/AIDS Policy, 1994–2004: How Can It Be Explained?', *African Affairs* 105(417): 591–614.
Butler, J. (1999) *Gender Trouble: Feminism and the Subversion of Identity*. London: Routledge.
Cameron, E. (2005) *Witness to AIDS*. Cape Town: Tafelberg.
Campbell, C. and Williams, B. (1999) 'Riding the Tiger: Contextualizing HIV Prevention in South Africa', *African Affairs* 100: 135–140.
CDC (Centers for Disease Control and Prevention) (2006) 'HIV/AIDS Basics', at: www.cdc.gov/hiv/resources/qa/definitions.htm (accessed 23 January 2013).
Césaire, A. (1955) *Discourse on Colonialism*. London: Monthly Review Press.
Chigwedere, P., Seage, G., Gruskin, S., Tun-Hou, L. and Essex, M. (2008) 'Estimating the Lost Benefits of Antiretroviral Drug Use in South Africa', *Journal of Acquired Immune Deficiency Syndrome* 2008: 1–6.
Clayden, P., Sharp, M. and TAC activists (2013) *HIV in Our Lives: Information for People Living with HIV/AIDS, Their Support Groups and Clinics*, at: www.tac.org.za/sites/default/files/publications/2014-10-31/TAC_IOL_web3_LR-1.pdf (accessed 26 January 2015).
Colvin, C. J., Robins, S. and Leavens, J. (2010) 'Grounding "Responsibilisation Talk": Masculinities, Citizenship and HIV in Cape Town, South Africa', *Journal of Development Studies* 46(7): 1179–1195.
Conrad, P. (1992) 'Medicalization and Social Control', *Annual Review of Sociology* 18: 209–232.
Coole, D. and Frost, S. (2010) 'Introducing the New Materialisms', in Coole, D. and Frost, S. (eds) *New Materialisms: Ontology, Agency and Politics*. Durham, NC: Duke University Press, pp. 1–43.
Craddock, S. (2004) 'Introduction: Beyond Epidemiology: Locating AIDS in Africa', in Kalipeni, E., Craddock, S., Oppong, J. R. et al. (eds) *HIV and AIDS in Africa: Beyond Epidemiology*. Malden, MA: Blackwell, pp. 1–10.
Crush, J. and Tawodzera, G. (2011) *Medical Xenophobia: Zimbabwean Access to Health Services in South Africa*. Migration Policy Series, 54, at: http://www.queensu.ca/samp/sampresources/samppublications/policyseries/Acrobat54.pdf (accessed 28 November 2012).

Crush, J. and Williams, V. (2001) 'Making Up the Numbers: Measuring "Illegal Immigration" to South Africa', Migration Policy Brief No. 3, at: http://www.queensu.ca/samp/sampresources/samppublications/policybriefs/brief3.pdf (accessed 6 December 2012).

Curry, E. (2011) 'New, Assertive Women's Voices in Local Elections', Inter Press Service News Agency, at: www.ipsnews.net/2011/01/south-africa-new-assertive-womens-voices-in-local-elections/ (accessed 15 June 2012).

de Paoli, M. M., Grønningsæter, A. B. and Mills, E. (2010) 'HIV/AIDS, the Disability Grant and ARV Adherence: Summary report', Fafo report 28, at www.fafo.no/pub/rapp/20172/20172.pdf (accessed 24 April 2012).

Decoteau, C. (2008) *The Bio-politics of HIV/AIDS in Post-apartheid South Africa*. PhD thesis, University of Michigan, Ann Arbor.

Decoteau, C. (2013) *Ancestors and Antiretrovirals: The Biopolitics of HIV/AIDS in South Africa*. Chicago: University of Chicago Press.

Department of Health (2012) The National Strategic Plan on HIV, STIs and TB (2012–2016), at www.hst.org.za/sites/default/files/hiv_nsp.pdf (accessed 31 July 2014).

Derrida, J. (1982) *Margins of Philosophy*. Chicago: University of Chicago Press.

Dolphijn, R. and van der Tuin, I. (2012) *New Materialism: Interviews and Cartographies*. Ann Arbor: Open Humanities Press.

Durban Declaration: A Declaration by Scientists and Physicians Affirming HIV is the Cause of AIDS (2000) *Nature* 406: 15–16.

Edge, D. (1995) 'Reinventing the Wheel', in Jasanoff, S., Markle, G., Peterson, J. et al. (eds) *Handbook of Science and Technology Studies*. London: Sage, pp. 3–23.

Epstein, S. (1996) *Impure Science: AIDS, Activism and the Politics of Knowledge*. Berkeley: University of California Press.

Fanon, F. (1967a) *Black Skin, White Masks*. New York: Grove Press.

Fanon, F. (1967b) *The Wretched of the Earth*. Harmondsworth: Penguin.

Fassin, D. (2007) *When Bodies Remember: Experiences and Politics of AIDS in South Africa*. Berkeley: University of California Press.

Fee, E. and Krieger, N. (1993) 'Understanding AIDS: Historical Interpretations and the Limits of Biomedical Individualism', *American Journal of Public Health* 83(10): 1477–1486.

Foucault, M. (1973) *The Birth of the Clinic: An Archaeology of Medical Perception*. London: Routledge.

Foucault, M. (2003) *'Society Must Be Defended': Lectures at the Collège de France 1975–76*. New York: Picador.

Fourie, P. and Meyer, M. (2010) *The Politics of AIDS Denialism: South Africa's Failure to Respond*. Aldershot: Ashgate.

Fraser, S. (2006) 'The Chronotope of the Queue: Methadone Maintenance Treatment and the Production of Time, Space and Subjects', *International Journal of Drug Policy* 17: 192–202.

Fraser, S. and Moore, D. (2008) 'Dazzled by Unity? Order and Chaos in Public Discourse on Illicit Drug Use', *Social Science & Medicine* 66(3): 740–752.

Fraser, S. and Seear, K. (2011) *Making Disease, Making Citizens: The Politics of Hepatitis C*. Aldershot: Ashgate.

Fuss, D. (1996) 'Introduction: Human, All Too Human', in Fuss, D. (ed.) *Human All Too Human*. London: Routledge, pp. 1–7.

Geffen, N. (2005) 'Echoes of Lysenko: State-sponsored Pseudo-science in South Africa', *Social Dynamics: A Journal of African Studies* 31(2): 183–210.

Geffen, N. (2006) 'How We Know that HIV Causes AIDS', *Equal Treatment*, March, at: www.tac.org.za (accessed 18 March 2011).

Geffen, N. (2010) *Debunking Delusions: The Inside Story of the Treatment Action Campaign.* Johannesburg: Jacana Media.

Gevisser, M. (2009) *A Legacy of Liberation: Thabo Mbeki and the Future of the South African Dream.* New York: Palgrave Macmillan.

Gieryn, T. (1995) 'Boundaries of Science', in Jasanoff, S., Markle, G., Peterson, J. et al. (eds) *Handbook of Science and Technology Studies.* London: Sage, pp. 393–443.

Gieryn, T. (1999) *Cultural Boundaries of Science: Credibility on the Line.* Chicago: University of Chicago Press.

Gumede, W. (2005) *Thabo Mbeki and the Battle for the Soul of the ANC.* Cape Town: Zebra Press.

Guy, R., McDonald, A., Bartlett, M., Murray, J., Giele, C., Davey, T. et al. (2007) 'HIV Diagnoses in Australia: Diverging Epidemics within a Low-prevalence Country', *Medical Journal of Australia* 187(8): 437–440.

Haraway, D. (1989) *Primate Visions: Gender, Race and Nature in the World of Modern Science.* New York: Routledge.

Haraway, D. (1991) *Simians, Cyborgs, and Women: The Reinvention of Nature.* London: Routledge.

Harding, S. (1986) *The Science Question in Feminism.* Ithaca, NY: Cornell University Press.

Harding, S. (1991) *Whose Science? Whose Knowledge? Thinking from Women's Lives.* Ithaca, NY: Cornell University Press.

Harris, B., Goudge, J., Ataguba, J. E., McIntyre, D., Nxumalo N., Jikwana, S. et al. (2011) 'Inequities in Access to Health Care in South Africa', *Journal of Public Health Policy* 32(S1): 102–123.

Hartley, W. (2001) 'State Boosts AIDS Spending', *Business Day*, at: www.hst.org.za/news/state-boosts-aids-spending (accessed 21 November 2012).

Heywood, M. (2003) 'Preventing Mother-to-Child HIV Transmission in South Africa: Background, Strategies and Outcomes of the Treatment Action Campaign Case against the Minister of Health', *South African Journal on Human Rights* 19: 278–315.

Heywood, M. (2004) 'The Price of Denial', at: www.tac.org.za/Documents/PriceOfDenial.doc (accessed 18 April 2013).

Heywood, M. (2005) 'The Achilles Heel? The Impact of HIV/AIDS on Democracy in South Africa', in Abdool Karim, S. and Abdool Karim, Q. (eds) *HIV/AIDS in South Africa.* Cambridge: Cambridge University Press, pp. 371–383.

Hodes, R. (2011) '"We Are the Loudmouthed HIV-Positive People! *Siyayinqoba/Beat It!*" on South African Television', in Barz, G. and Cohan, J. M. (eds) *The Culture of AIDS in Africa: Hope and Healing through Music and the Arts.* Oxford: Oxford University Press, pp. 158–179.

Human Rights Watch (2008) 'Neighbors in Need: Zimbabweans Seeking Refuge in South Africa', at: www.hrw.org/sites/default/files/reports/southafrica0608_1.pdf (accessed 5 December 2012).

International AIDS Society (IAS) (2009) 'Fact Sheet: HIV/AIDS in sub-Saharan Africa and South Africa', paper delivered at the 5th International Conference on HIV Pathogenesis, Treatment and Prevention, Cape Town, South Africa, 19–22 July.
Jensen, T. E. and Winthereik, B. R. (2005) 'Review of *The Body Multiple: Ontology in Medical Practice*', *Acta Sociologica* 48(3): 266–268.
Jones, P. (2009) *AIDS Treatment and Human Rights in Context*. New York: Palgrave.
Kalichman, S. C. (2009) *Denying AIDS: Conspiracy Theories, Pseudoscience and Human Tragedy*. New York: Copernicus Books.
Kapczynski, A. and Berger, J. M. (2009) 'The Story of the TAC Case: The Potential and Limits of Socio-economic Rights Litigation in South Africa', *Human Rights Advocacy Stories*, at: www.law.berkeley.edu/php-programs/faculty/facultyPubsPDF.php?facID=7238&pubID=2 (accessed 12 November 2012).
Kapp, C. (2006) 'South African Health Minister Must Go, Say Scientists', *The Lancet* 368(9542): 1141–1142.
Karavanta, M. and Morgan, N. (2008) 'Introduction: "Humanism, Hybridity and Democratic Praxis"', in Karavanta, M. and Morgan, N. (eds) *Edward Said and Jacques Derrida: Reconstellating Humanism and the Global Hybrid*. Cambridge: Cambridge Scholars Publishing, pp. 1–23.
Keller, E. F. (1985) *Reflections on Gender and Science*. New Haven, CT: Yale University Press.
Keller, E. F. (1995) ' "Gender and Science": A First Person Account', in Jasanoff, S., Markle, G., Peterson, J. et al. (eds) *The Handbook of Science and Technology Studies*. London: Sage, pp. 80–94.
King, R. (1999) 'Sexual Behavioural Change for HIV: Where Have Theories Taken Us?', Joint United Nations Programme on HIV/AIDS (UNAIDS), at: www.who.int/hiv/strategic/surveillance/en/unaids_99_27.pdf (accessed 10 October 2011).
Kirby, V. (2008) 'Natural Convers(at)ions: Or What If Culture Was Really Nature All Along?', in Alaimo, S. and Hekman, S. (eds) *Material Feminisms*. Bloomington: Indiana University Press, pp. 214–236.
Kirby, V. (2011) *Quantum Anthropologies: Life at Large*. Durham, NC: Duke University Press.
Kleine, M. (1994) 'Metaphor and the Discourse of Virology: HIV as Human Being', *Journal of Medical Humanities* 15(2): 123–139.
Kumar, M. P. (2011) '(An)other Way of Being Human: "Indigenous" Alternative(s) to Postcolonial Humanism', *Third World Quarterly* 32(9): 1557–1572.
Latour, B. (2004) 'Why Has Critique Run Out of Steam? From Matters of Fact to Matters of Concern', *Critical Inquiry* 30: 225–248.
Leclerc-Madlala, S. (2006) ' "We Will Eat When I Get the Grant": Negotiating AIDS, Poverty and Antiretroviral Treatment in South Africa', *African Journal of AIDS Research* 5(3): 249–256.
Lezaun, J. (2014) 'A Reader's Guide to the "Ontological Turn" – Part 2', *Somatosphere*, at: http://somatosphere.net/2014/01/a-readers-guide-to-the-ontological-turn-part-2.html (accessed 14 February 2014).
Lock, M. and Nguyen, V.-K. (2010) *An Anthropology of Biomedicine*. Chichester: Wiley Blackwell.

Bibliography

Low, M. (2009) 'Quackery Is All Around Us', December, at: www.tac.org.za (accessed 22 August 2011).

Low, M., Tomlinson, C., Kardas-Nelson, M., Kim, K. and Geffen, N. (2010) *Fighting for Our Lives: The History of the Treatment Action Campaign (1998–2010)*. Cape Town: Treatment Action Campaign.

Lupton, D. (1997) 'Foucault and the Medicalisation Critique', in Peterson, A. and Bunton, R. (eds) *Foucault, Health and Medicine*. London: Routledge, pp. 94–112.

Makgoba, M. (2000) 'HIV/AIDS: The Peril of Pseudoscience', *Science*, 288(5469): 1171.

Makgoba, M. (2002) 'Politics, the Media and Science in HIV/AIDS: The Peril of Pseudoscience', *Vaccine* 20(15): 1899–1904.

Maqungo, B. (2001) Affidavit, at: www.tac.org.za/Documents/MTCTCourtCase/ccmbusi.txt (accessed 7 December 2014).

Marais, H. (2005) 'Buckling: The Impact of AIDS in South Africa', at: http://gametlibrary.worldbank.org/FILES/317_The impact of AIDS in South Africa_Research Report.pdf (accessed 10 August 2012).

Marcus, G. and Shaskalson, M. (2001) *Pharmaceutical Manufacturers Association (PMA) and Others v the President of the Republic of South Africa and Others and the Treatment Action Campaign (Amicus Curaie)*. Bloemfontein: Transvaal Provinical Court.

Marcus, G. and Majola, B. (2001) *TAC and Others v Minister of Health and Others*. Bloemfontein: Transvaal Provincial Division of the High Court of South Africa.

Martin, E. (1996) 'The Egg and the Sperm: How Science Has Constructed a Romance Based on Stereotypical Male–Female Roles', in Fox Keller, E. and Longino, H. (eds) *Feminism and Science*. Oxford: Oxford University Press, pp. 103–117.

Maurice, J. (2014) 'South Africa's Battle against HIV/AIDS Gains Momentum', *Lancet*, 383(9928): 1535–1536.

Mbali, M. (2004) 'AIDS Discourses and the South African State: Government Denialism and Post-apartheid AIDS Policy-making', *Transformation* 54: 104–120.

Mbali, M. (2013) *South African AIDS Activism and Global Health Politics*. Basingstoke: Palgrave Macmillan.

Mbeki, T. (2000a) 'Health, Human Dignity, and Partners for Poverty Reduction', *ANC Today*, 2, at: www.anc.org.za/docs/anctoday/2002/at14.htm (accessed 4 April 2011).

Mbeki, T. (2000b) 'Letter from Mbeki to Tony Leon (dated 1 July 2000)', *Sunday Times*, at: www.virusmyth.com/aids/news/letmbeki.htm (accessed 20 March 2011).

Mbeki, T. (2000c) 'Letter to World Leaders on AIDS in Africa (dated 3 April 2000)', at: http://tmh.floonet.net/articles/mbeki.shtml (accessed 10 May 2010).

Mbeki, T. (2000d) Speech of the President of South Africa, Thabo Mbeki, at the opening session of the 13th International AIDS Conference, at: www.virusmyth.com/aids/news/durbspmbeki.htm (accessed 31 January 2013).

Mbeki, T. (2001) 'Transcript of e-TV Interview with Debora Patta', 24 April, at: www.virusmyth.com/aids/news/etvmbeki.htm (accessed 28 June 2011).

Mbeki, T. (2004a) 'Dislodging Stereotypes', *ANC Today*, 4, at: www.anc.org.za/docs/anctoday/2004/at42.html (accessed 29 March 2011).

Mbeki, T. (2004b) 'When Is Good News Bad News?', *ANC Today*, 4, at: www.anc.org.za/docs/anctoday/2004/at39.htm (accessed 13 April 2011).
Memmi, A. (1990) *The Colonizer and the Colonized*. London: Earthscan.
Mol, A. (1999) 'Ontological Politics: A Word and Some Questions', *Sociological Review* 46: 74–89.
Mol, A. (2002) *The Body Multiple: Ontology in Medical Practice*. Durham, NC: Duke University Press.
Mol, A. and Berg, M. (1998) *Differences in Medicine: Unraveling Practices, Techniques, and Bodies*. Durham, NC: Duke University Press.
Mol, A. and Law, J. (2002) 'Complexities: An Introduction', in Law, J. and Mol, A. (eds) *Complexities: Social Studies of Knowledge Practices*. Durham, NC: Duke University Press, pp. 1–21.
Mol, A. and Law, J. (2004) 'Embodied Action, Enacted Bodies: The Example of Hypoglycaemia', *Body & Society* 10(2–3): 43–62.
Montaner, J. (2011) 'Treatment as Prevention – A Double Hat-Trick', *Lancet* 378(9787): 208– 209.
Mthathi, S. (2006) 'Editorial: Science and Human Rights', *Equal Treatment*, March, at: www.tac.org.za (accessed 18 March 2011).
Mykhalovskiy, E. and Rosengarten, M. (2009) 'HIV/AIDS in its Third Decade: Renewed Critique in Social and Cultural Analysis – An Introduction', *Social Theory and Health* 7(3): 187–195.
National Antenatal Sentinel HIV and Syphilis Prevalence Survey (2008) *South Africa Report*, at: www.doh.gov.za/docs/reports/2009/nassps/index.html (accessed 19 April 2010).
Nguyen, V., Bajos N., Dubois-Arber, F., O'Malley, J. and Pirkle, C. M. (2011) 'Remedicalizing an Epidemic: From HIV Treatment as Prevention to HIV Treatment is Prevention', *AIDS* 25(3): 291–293.
Oppenheimer, G. (1988) 'In the Eye of the Storm: The Epidemiological Construcion of AIDS', in Fee, E. and Fox, D. (eds) *AIDS: The Burdens of History*. Berkeley: University of California Press, pp. 267–300.
Otto, D. (1997) 'Rethinking the "Universality" of Human Rights Law', *Columbia Human Rights Law Review* 29: 1–46.
Parliament of the Republic of South Africa (2000) Proceedings of the National Assembly, 5 April, at: www.parliament.gov.za/live/commonrepository/Processed/20110729/92607_1.doc (accessed 1 March 2015).
Parliament of the Republic of South Africa (2004) National Assembly Executive Replies to Questions, at: www.pmg.org.za (accessed 31 January 2015).
Patterson, A. S. (2006) *The Politics of AIDS in Africa*. Boulder, CO: Lynne Rienner.
Patton, C. (1990) *Inventing AIDS*. New York: Routledge.
Peacock, D., Budaza, T. and Greig, A. (2007) ' "Justice for Lorna Mlofana": The Treatment Action Campaign's AIDS and Gender Activism', in Ndinga-Muvumba, A. (ed.) *From Moralizing to Preventive Action: HIV/AIDS and Human Security in South Africa*. Cape Town: Centre for Conflict Resolution.
Peacock, D., Budaza, T. and Greig, A. (2008) 'The Treatment Action Campaign's Activism', in Ndinga-Muvumba, A. and Pharaoh, R. (eds) *HIV/AIDS and Society in South Africa*. Scottsville: University of KwaZulu-Natal Press, pp. 85–102.
Persson, A. (2013) 'Non/infectious Corporealities: Tensions in the Biomedical Era of "HIV Normalisation" ', *Sociology of Health & Illness* 35(7): 1065–1079.

Petersen, A., Davis, M., Fraser, S. and Lindsay, J. (2010) 'Healthy Living and Citizenship: An Overview', *Critical Public Health* 20(4): 391–400.
Posel, D. (2005) 'Sex, Death and the Fate of the Nation: Reflections on the Politicization of Sexuality in Post-Apartheid South Africa', *Africa: Journal of the International African Institute* 75(2): 125–153.
Race, K. (2001) 'The Undetectable Crisis: Changing Technologies of Risk', *Sexualities* 4(2): 167–189.
Race, K. (2012) 'Framing Responsibility HIV, Biomedical Prevention, and the Performativity of the Law', *Journal of Bioethical Inquiry* 9(3): 327–338.
Ramatlhodi, N., Mbeki, T., Pahad, E. and Gumbi, M. (2000) Letter to Professor William Makgoba (dated 11 December 2000), at: www.politicsweb.co.za (accessed 30 August 2011).
Ramphele, M. (2001) 'Citizenship Challenges for South Africa's Young Democracy', *Daedalus* 130(1): 1–17.
Republic of South Africa (1996) The Bill of Rights of the Constitution of the Republic of South Africa, *Government Gazette*, No. 108, at: www.info.gov.za/documents/constitution/1996/96cons2.htm (accessed 11 October 2012).
Robins, S. (2006) 'From "Rights" to "Ritual": AIDS Activism in South Africa', *American Anthropologist*, 108: 312–323.
Robins, S. (2009) 'Foot Soldiers of Global Health: Teaching and Preaching AIDS Science and Modern Medicine on the Frontline', *Medical Anthropology* 28(1): 81–107.
Robins, S. and von Lieres, B. (2004) 'Remaking Citizenship, Unmaking Marginalization: The Treatment Action Campaign in Post-Apartheid South Africa', *Canadian Journal of African Studies* 38(3): 575–585.
Rose, N. (2007) *The Politics of Life Itself: Biomedicine, Power, and Subjectivity in the Twenty-First Century*. Princeton, NJ: Princeton University Press.
Rose, N. and Novas, C. (2005) 'Biological Citizenship', in Ong, A. and Collier, S. J. (eds) *Global Assemblages: Technology, Politics and Ethics as Anthropological Problems*. Malden, MA: Blackwell, pp. 439–463.
Rosengarten, M. (2009) *HIV Interventions: Biomedicine and the Traffic between Information and Flesh*. Seattle: University of Washington Press.
Rosengarten, M. and Michael, M. (2009) 'Rethinking the Bioethical Enactment of Medically Drugged Bodies: Paradoxes of Using Anti-HIV Drug Therapy as Technology for Prevention', *Science as Culture* 18(2): 183–199.
Roux, N. L. and Nyamukachi, P. (2005) 'A Reform Model for the Improvement of Municipal Service Delivery in South Africa', *Journal of Public Administration*, Special Issue 3 40: 687–705.
Schneider, H. (2002) 'On the Fault-line: The Politics of AIDS Policy in Contemporary South Africa', *African Studies* 21(1): 145–167.
Schneider, H. and Fassin, D. (2002) 'Denial and Defiance: A Socio-political Analysis of AIDS in South Africa', *AIDS* 16(4): 45–50.
Seear, K. (2014) *The Makings of a Modern Epidemic: Endometriosis, Gender and Culture*. Aldershot: Ashgate.
Setiloane, T. (2012) 'Beyond Advocacy – Business Needs to Get in Ahead of the Game', *McKinsey on Society*, at: http://voices.mckinseyonsociety.com/south-africa-unemployment-in-youth/ (accessed 14 March 2013).
Shah, S. (2006) *The Body Hunters: Testing New Drugs on the World's Poorest Patients*. New York: New Press.

Shapurjee, Y. and Charlton, S. (2013) 'Transforming South Africa's Low-income Housing Projects through Backyard Dwellings: Intersections with Households and the State in Alexandra, Johannesburg', *Journal of Housing and the Built Environment* 28(4): 653–666.

Shisana, O. and Simbayi, L. (2002) 'Nelson Mandela HSRC Study of HIV/AIDS: South African National HIV Prevalence, Behavioural Risks and Mass Media Household Survey', at: www.wsu.ac.za/hsrc/html/2007-2.pdf (accessed 26 July 2012).

Shisana, O., Rehle, T., Simbayi, L.C., Zuma, K., Jooste, S., Zungu, N. *et al.* (2014) *South African National HIV Prevalence, Incidence and Behaviour Survey, 2012*. Cape Town: HSRC Press.

Singer, M. (2004) 'The Social Origins and Expressions of Illness', *British Medical Bulletin* 69(1): 9–16.

Singer, M. and Baer, H. (2007) *Introducing Medical Anthropology: A Discipline in Action*. Lanham, MD: Altamira Press.

South African HIV Clinicians Society (2012) 'Guidance to Clinicians Experiencing Tenofovir and Abacavir Drug Shortages', at: http://www.tac.org.za/community/node/3273 (accessed 23 May 2012).

South African National Aids Council (2007) *HIV and AIDS and STI Strategic Plan for South Africa 2007–2011*, at: www.womensnet.org.za/services/NSP/NSP-2007-2011-Draft9.pdf (accessed 21 April 2010).

Statistics South Africa (2010) 'Monthly Earnings of South Africans, 2010 (Quarterly Labour Force Survey)', at: www.statssa.gov.za/publications/P02112/P021122010.pdf (accessed 7 June 2013).

Swanson, M. W. (1977) 'The Sanitation Syndrome: Bubonic Plague and Urban Native Policy in the Cape Colony, 1900–1909', *Journal of African History* 18(3): 387–410.

TAC (2001) 'MTCP Court Case Victory! (TAC press release dated 14 Dec 2001)', at: www.tac.org.za/newsletter/2001/ns14_12_2001.txt (accessed 1 March 2015).

TAC (2009) 'Landmark Speech by President Zuma', at: www.tac.org.za/news/landmark-speech-president-zuma-0 (accessed 12 July 2015).

TAC (2012) 'Civil Society Organisations Call for an Enquiry into the Ongoing Stock-outs of Medicines', *TAC Electronic Newsletter*, at: www.tac.org.za (accessed 23 May 2012).

TAC authors (2012) 'HIV Life Cycle: How the Virus Multiplies Inside Our Bodies', *Equal Treatment: Magazine of the Treatment Action Campaign* 42(April).

TAC contributors (2006) *ARVs in Our Lives: A Handbook for People Living with HIV and Treatment Advocates in Support Groups, Clinics and Communities*, at: www.tac.org.za./sites/default/files/publications/2012-09-27/arvsinourlives.pdf (accessed 31 January 2015).

TAC Science and Research Committee (2001) 'Draft Discussion Document: Integrated Framework for a National HIV/AIDS Treatment and Prevention Plan', in *The Zackie Achmat, Jack Lewis and Treatment Action Campaign Political Papers*. Johannesburg: University of the Witwatersrand's Historical Papers Library.

TAC writer (2012) 'Immediate Action Required to Solve the Systemic Crisis at Mthatha Medical Depot and to Save Patients' Lives', at: www.tac.org.za/news/immediate-action-required-solve-systemic-crisis-mthatha-medical-depot-and-save-patients%D5-lives (accessed 3 December 2012).

Tladi, L. (2006) 'Poverty and HIV/AIDS in South Africa: An Empirical Contribution', *Journal of Social Aspects of HIV/AIDS* 3(1): 369–381.
Treichler, P. (1999) *How to Have Theory in an Epidemic: Cultural Chronicles of AIDS*. Durham, NC: Duke University Press.
Tshabalala-Msimang, M. (2004) 'An Accessible, Caring and High Quality Health System', *ANC Today*, 4, at: www.anc.org.za/docs/anctoday/2004/at30.htm – art1 (accessed 29 March 2011).
UNAIDS (2012) 'HIV and AIDS Estimates', at: www.unaids.org/en/regionscountries/countries/southafrica/ (accessed 11 December 2013).
van der Vliet, V. (2004) 'South Africa Divided against AIDS: A Crisis of Leadership', in Kauffman, K. and Lindauer, D. (eds) *AIDS and South Africa: The Social Expression of a Pandemic*. Basingstoke: Palgrave Macmillan, pp. 48–96.
Vasudev, N. (2008) 'Income or Health: Can HIV Patients Have Both?', *Oxfam News E-Magazine (O.N.E.)* August (Hong Kong, Oxfam International).
Vitellone, N. (2011) 'Contesting Compassion', *Sociological Review* 59(3): 579–596.
Waldby, C. (1996) *AIDS and the Body Politic: Biomedicine and Sexual Difference*. London: Routledge.
Wang, J. (2004) 'AIDS Denialism and "The Humanisation of the African"', *Race & Class* 49(3): 1–18.
WebMD (2012) 'HIV, AIDS, and the CD4 Count', *Web MD Medical Reference*, at: www.webmd.com/hiv-aids/cd4-count-what-does-it-mean (accessed 24 January 2013).
Weiss, M. (1997) 'Signifying the Pandemics: Metaphors of AIDS, Cancer, and Heart Disease', *Medical Anthropology Quarterly* 11(4): 456–476.
Wood, K., Lambert, H. and Jewkes, R. (2007) ' "Showing Roughness in a Beautiful Way": Talk about Love, Coercion, and Rape in South African Youth Sexual Culture', *Medical Anthropology Quarterly* 21(3): 277–300.
WHO (World Health Organization) (2013) 'Antiretroviral Therapy', at www.who.int/topics/antiretroviral_therapy/en/ (accessed 23 January 2013).
Yeğenoğlu, M. (1998) *Colonial Fantasies: Towards a Feminist Reading of Orientalism*. Cambridge: Cambridge University Press.
Youdé, J. (2005) 'The Development of a Counter-epistemic Community: AIDS, South Africa and International Regimes', *International Relations* 19(4): 421–439.
Youdé, J. (2007a) *AIDS, South Africa and the Politics of Knowledge*. Aldershot: Ashgate.
Youdé, J. (2007b) 'Ideology's Role in AIDS Policies in Uganda and South Africa', *Global Health Governance* 1(January): 1–16.
Zuma, J. (2009) Address by the President of the Republic of South Africa, HE Mr Jacob Zuma, to the National Council of Provinces (NCOP), at: www.thepresidency.gov.za/pebble.asp?relid=595 (accessed 12 July 2015).

Index

Achmat, Z., 135, 136, 138
African nationalism, 49, 97–8, 100
agential cut, 51, 52, 60, 143n10, 143n11
agential realism, 12, 24, 29–31, 33–4, 63, 65, 124
Angelides, S., 89
anti-retroviral drugs (ARVs)
  access to, 12–13, 19, 63, 72, 74, 77–8, 83–4, 87, 102, 104, 109, 114
  and adherence, 78, 113–15, 118, 120, 129, 131–2, 143n4
  decoupling of HIV and AIDS through, 87, 111, 141n1
  dosing regimes of, 62, 75, 89, 118
  generative role of, 75–6, 120
  side-effects of, 115, 120, 129
  and treatment-as-prevention, 59, 62
  and viral resistance, 62, 78, 114, 129
agency
  agential realism on, 12, 29, 32
  in calculations of sexual risk, 80–1
  of matter, 32
AIDS, see also HIV, 111–12, 141n1
  decoupling of HIV from, 87, 111, 141n1
  dissidence, 3–4, 6–9, 52, 64, 86, 96–8, 104, 124
  apartheid and racial oppression, 41–2, 47–50, 64, 110–11, 117, 124, 125
Australia, HIV in, 79

Bacchi, C., 59, 130
Barad, K., 12, 22, 23, 25, 29, 30, 32–3, 40, 52, 53, 54, 61, 72, 99–100, 104, 121, 129, 130, 133–4, 142n2, 143n11
binary oppositions, see also dualisms, 16, 17, 18, 20–2, 30, 56–7, 59–61, 63, 65, 67–8, 70–3, 92, 93–4, 96–7, 101, 123–4, 126, 128, 131

biological citizenship, 18, 88–91, 107–16, 117, 127–8
biopower, 88, 91, 117
Butler, J., 30

Cameron, E., 9, 49, 101
CD4 cells, 21–2, 31–2, 142n1
  CD4 count, 109
civil disobedience, 4, 138
common-sense realism, 33, 45
condoms, role in HIV prevention, see also prevention, 10, 53, 60, 61, 65, 70, 71, 87, 130, 132, 140
conflict, over science of HIV, see also struggles over science, 2–5, 11, 20, 27, 32, 65, 74, 135–40
Craddock, S., 47, 64

Decoteau, C., 72–3, 88, 110
disease
  intra-activity of, 29–32, 53–4, 62, 64, 72–3, 75–9, 104, 118–19, 132–3
  medico-scientific accounts of, 25, 32
  as ontologically multiple, 26–7, 54, 70, 111–12, 115–16, 117, 121–2, 127, 134
  social constructivist accounts of, 25
  dissidence, 3–5, 6–9, 64, 96–8, 104
  drug-resistant virus, 31–2, 62, 75, 78, 114, 120, 129
dualisms, see also binary oppositions, 16, 17, 18, 20–2, 30, 56–7, 59–61, 63, 65, 67–8, 70–3, 92, 93–4, 96–7, 101, 123–4, 126, 128, 131

epidemiology, role in shaping HIV, 103–4, 130–1
Epstein, S., 44

Fanon, F., 98, 144n1, 144n2
Fassin, D., 6, 46, 49, 50, 137, 143n9

feminist approaches, 5, 22–3, 29–30, 44, 106, 142n4
Foucault, M., 52, 112, 129
Fraser, S., 7, 29, 35, 63, 89, 112–13, 141n5
Fuss, D., 98, 99

Gay Related Immune Deficiency (GRID), 102–3
Geffen, N., 1, 53, 73–7, 135, 142n3
gender
  performativity of, 30
  in vulnerability to HIV, 37, 39–40, 64, 87, 100, 116, 132, 142n1
gender-based violence, role in South Africa's HIV epidemic, 37, 39–40, 64, 87, 100, 132, 142n1
genealogy, 8, 46–50
Gieryn, T., *see also* science, boundary-work of, 16, 54–5, 57, 143n11

Haraway, D., 23, 142n4
highly active anti-retroviral therapy, *see also* anti-retroviral drugs (ARVs), 19, 141n2, 142n1, 144n4
HIV
  clinical trials, 58–9
  decoupling of AIDS from, 87, 111, 141n1
  definition of, 241n1
  infection rates of, 2, 102, 103
  life cycle of, 21–2
  mortality, 2, 72–3, 102, 104, 125, 130
  ontologies of, 103–4, 111–12, 115–16, 117, 127
  poverty in the making of, 17, 31–2, 63, 64, 73–80, 83, 94, 116, 124, 125, 131
  prevalence in South Africa, 39–40, 80, 102–4, 140
  prevention, 4, 60–1, 84–7, 105–6, 108, 132, 137
  science of, 9, 21–4
  viral mutation of, 32, 62, 75, 78, 120

women's vulnerability to, 10, 37–41, 46
human rights, 104–9, 111–12, 116, 128
humanism, 18, 96, 98–100, 112, 115, 116–17, 124, 142n2, 144n2

interventions, generative role of, 10–11, 24, 62, 75–6, 80
intra-action, 12, 24, 29–32, 40, 53–4, 62, 72–3, 75–9, 104, 118–19, 121, 123, 125, 132–3

Latour, B., 28–9, 32–3, 36, 59, 60, 66, 121
Law, J., 26, 27, 141n3

Martin, E., 23, 44, 142n4
material determinism, 15–6, 25–6
matters of concern, 28–9, 32–4, 60, 66, 104, 121, 131
matters of fact, 10, 11–12, 19, 28–9, 33, 56–64, 65–6, 104, 121, 123–4, 130–1
Mbeki, T.
  critique of HIV science, 35–6, 44–5, 50–1, 59–60, 64, 100–1, 135
  on racism, 35–46, 96–8, 100–2, 125
  on relationship between poverty and HIV, 17, 68, 79, 81–3, 92
  medicalisation, 62, 70–2, 77–8
Michael, M., 58–9, 75–6
Mol, A., 10–11, 15, 25–7, 33, 121–2, 133, 141n3

neoliberal subjects
new materialisms, 12, 32, 141n4

ontological politics, 11–12, 133, 141n3
ontologies
  and multiplicity, 26–7, 54, 70
  as co-constituted, 22–3, 54, 70, 78
  as emergent and open-ended, 5, 9–12, 19, 78
  of disease, 5, 6–8, 9–12, 15–16, 19, 24–7, 31, 54, 70, 78
Oppenheimer, G., 103

parliamentary debate, analysis of, 36–43
people living with HIV, 17–18, 126
  as biological citizens, 87–91, 97, 107–16, 127
  as 'disease vectors', 79–80, 81–2, 92, 101
  as 'victims', 79–80, 81–2, 84–6, 92
performativity, 7, 15, 20, 22, 26, 30, 32, 45–6, 101, 102–3, 116, 126, 128–30, 141n4, 143n11
phenomenon, agential realist concept of, 32–3
policy
  role in shaping HIV, 31, 80–1, 94–5, 129–30
  of South Africa on HIV, 105, 139, 140
post-humanism, 5, 12, 16, 80–1, 91, 113, 133–4
  in challenging norms of biological citizenship, 113, 115, 117–18, 127–9
  in rethinking human/non-human binary, 22–4, 99–100
poverty, in the making of HIV, 17, 31–2, 63, 64, 73–9, 82
praxiography, 10, 26
prevention, see also HIV
  of mother-to-child transmission (PMTCT), 4, 84–7, 105–6, 108, 137
  role of condoms in, 10, 53, 60, 61, 65, 70, 71, 87, 130, 132, 140
Pre-Exposure Prophylaxis (PrEP), 58
pseudo-science, 9, 43, 51, 52–3, 96, 135, 139,
public health, role in shaping HIV, 41–2, 47–9, 61, 72–3, 80–1, 101, 104, 111–15, 118, 125, 126, 127–8, 129–30, 132

queer theory, 23

Race, K., 80, 89, 109–10, 114, 133
race, in conceptions of HIV, 46–50, 100–2

relationality, 12, 54, 69–70, 73, 76, 79–81, 93, 120, 123
representationalism, 25–6
Rose, N., 88, 90, 107, 117, 126, 129
Rosengarten, M., 7, 13, 22, 54, 58–9, 62, 63, 75, 80–1, 115, 118, 129

science
  boundary-work of, 16, 50–6
  of HIV, 9, 21–4
  struggles over, 2–5, 11, 20, 27, 32, 50–6, 65, 74, 135–40, see also conflict
Science and Technology Studies (STS), 5, 22–4
scientific realism, 36, 53
  critique of, 21–4, 25, 44, 53–4
Seear, K., 7, 29, 35, 63, 112–13, 141n5
sexual practices, and HIV transmission, 46–7, 65, 80, 81–3, 85–6, 87, 101
social constructivism, limitations of, 15–6, 25–6
South Africa
  history of HIV in, 2–5, 135–40
  HIV transmission rates in, 2
stigma, 7, 11, 29, 79, 81–3, 122, 126, 130–1, 136

Treatment Action Campaign (TAC)
  approach to HIV science, 51–6, 57, 73
  and HIV literacy, 87–91
  legal action of, 83–7, 105–6, 137, 144n3
  on relationship between poverty and HIV, 68–9, 73–7, 125
  and the struggle for HIV-treatment in South Africa, 83–7, 105–6, 137, 138, 144n3
Treichler, P., 6, 7, 47, 58
Tshabalala-Msimang, M., 3, 4, 52, 60–1, 135, 138, 139

viral load, 62, 78, 109–10

Waldby, C., 23–4, 91, 142n2, 142n3
Weiss, M., 22

The manufacturer's authorised representative in the EU is Springer Nature Customer Service Centre GmbH, Europaplatz 3, 69115 Heidelberg, Germany. If you have any concerns regarding our products, please contact ProductSafety@springernature.com

Printed and bound by CPI Group (UK) Ltd, Croydon, CR0 4YY

23/03/2026

02076402-0019